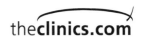

MEDICAL CLINICS

OF NORTH AMERICA

Pain Management, Part II

GUEST EDITOR
Howard S. Smith, MD

March 2007 • Volume 91 • Number 2

SAUNDERS

An Imprint of Elsevier, Inc.
PHILADELPHIA LONDON TORONTO MONTREAL SYDNEY TOKYO

W.B. SAUNDERS COMPANY
A Division of Elsevier Inc.

1600 John F. Kennedy Boulevard • Suite 1800 • Philadelphia, Pennsylvania 19103-2899

http://www.theclinics.com

MEDICAL CLINICS OF NORTH AMERICA   Volume 91, Number 2
March 2007   ISSN 0025-7125
Editor: Rachel Glover   ISBN-13: 978-1-4160-4780-3
     ISBN-10: 1-4160-4780-8

The ideas and opinions expressed in *Medical Clinics of North America* do not necessarily reflect those of the Publisher. The Publisher does not assume any responsibility for any injury and/or damage to persons or property arising out of or related to any use of the material contained in this periodical. The reader is advised to check the appropriate medical literature and the product information currently provided by the manufacturer of each drug to be administered to verify the dosage, the method and duration of administration, or contraindications. It is the responsibility of the treating physician or other health care professional, relying on independent experience and knowledge of the patient, to determine drug dosages and the best treatment for the patient. Mention of any product in this issue should not be construed as endorsement by the contributors, editors, or the Publisher of the product or manufacturers' claims.

Medical Clinics of North America (ISSN 0025-7125) is published bimonthly by W.B. Saunders, 360 Park Avenue South, New York, NY 10010-1710. Business and editorial offices: 1600 John F. Kennedy Boulevard, Suite 1800, Philadelphia, PA 19103-2899. Accounting and circulation offices: 6277 Sea Harbor Drive, Orlando, FL 32887-4800. Periodicals postage paid at New York, NY, and additional mailing offices. Subscription prices are USD 157 per year for US individuals, USD 273 per year for US institutions, USD 81 per year for US students, USD 200 per year for Canadian individuals, USD 347 per year for Canadian institutions, USD 119 per year for Canadian students, USD 227 per year for international individuals, USD 347 per year for international institutions and USD 119 per year for international students. To receive student/resident rate, orders must be accompanied by name of affiliated institution, date of term, and the *signature* of program/residency coordinator on institution letterhead. Orders will be billed at individual rate until proof of status is received. Foreign air speed delivery is included in all *Clinics* subscription prices. All prices are subject to change without notice. POSTMASTER: Send address changes to *Medical Clinics of North America*, Elsevier Periodicals Customer Service, 6277 Sea Harbor Drive, Orlando, FL 32887-4800. **Customer Service: 1-800-654-2452 (US). From outside of the USA, call (+1) 407-345-1000. E-mail: hhspcs@harcourt.com.**

Reprints. For copies of 100 or more, of articles in this publication, please contact the Commercial Reprints Department, Elsevier Inc., 360 Park Avenue South, New York, New York 10010-1710. Tel.: (+1) (212) 633-3813; Fax: (+1) (212) 462-1935; E-mail: reprints@elsevier.com.

Medical Clinics of North America is also published in Spanish by McGraw-Hill Interamericana Editores S. A., P.O. Box 5-237, 06500 Mexico, D.F., Mexico.

Medical Clinics of North America is covered in *Index Medicus, Current Contents, ASCA, Excerpta Medica, Science Citation Index,* and *ISI/BIOMED.*

Printed in the United States of America.

GOAL STATEMENT

The goal of *Medical Clinics of North America* is to keep practicing physicians up to date with current clinical practice by providing timely articles reviewing the state of the art in patient care.

ACCREDITATION

The *Medical Clinics of North America* is planned and implemented in accordance with the Essential Areas and Policies of the Accreditation Council for Continuing Medical Education (ACCME) through the joint sponsorship of the University of Virginia School of Medicine and Elsevier. The University of Virginia School of Medicine is accredited by the ACCME to provide continuing medical education for physicians.

The University of Virginia School of Medicine designates this educational activity for a maximum of 90 *AMA PRA Category 1 Credits*™. Physicians should only claim credit commensurate with the extent of their participation in the activity.

The American Medical Association has determined that physicians not licensed in the US who participate in this CME activity are eligible for *AMA PRA Category 1 Credits*™.

Credit can be earned by reading the text material, taking the CME examination online at http://www.theclinics.com/home/cme, and completing the evaluation. After taking the test, you will be required to review any and all incorrect answers. Following completion of the test and evaluation, your credit will be awarded and you may print your certificate.

FACULTY DISCLOSURE/CONFLICT OF INTEREST

The University of Virginia School of Medicine, as an ACCME accredited provider, endorses and strives to comply with the Accreditation Council for Continuing Medical Education (ACCME) Standards of Commercial Support, Commonwealth of Virginia statutes, University of Virginia policies and procedures, and associated federal and private regulations and guidelines on the need for disclosure and monitoring of proprietary and financial interests that may affect the scientific integrity and balance of content delivered in continuing medical education activities under our auspices.

The University of Virginia School of Medicine requires that all CME activities accredited through this institution be developed independently and be scientifically rigorous, balanced and objective in the presentation/discussion of its content, theories and practices.

All authors/editors participating in an accredited CME activity are expected to disclose to the readers relevant financial relationships with commercial entities occurring within the past 12 months (such as grants or research support, employee, consultant, stock holder, member of speakers bureau, etc.). The University of Virginia School of Medicine will employ appropriate mechanisms to resolve potential conflicts of interest to maintain the standards of fair and balanced education to the reader. Questions about specific strategies can be directed to the Office of Continuing Medical Education, University of Virginia School of Medicine, Charlottesville, Virginia.

The authors/editors listed below have identified no professional or financial affiliations for themselves or their spouse/partner:

Grace C. Chang, MD, MPH; Lucy Chen, MD; Anthony L. Dragovich, MD; Rachel Glover (Acquisitions Editor); Mohammed A. Khaleel, MS; Kenneth L. Kirsch, PhD; Lori Lavelle, DO; William Lavelle, MD; Elizabeth D. Lavelle, MD; Jianren Mao, MD, PhD; Gary McCleane, MD, FFARCSI; Annie G. Philip, MD; and, Howard S. Smith, MD (Guest Editor).

The authors/editors listed below identified the following professional or financial affiliations for themselves or their spouse/partner:

Allen Carl, MD is on the Advisory Committee for K2 Medical.
Steven P. Cohen, MD is funded in part by the John P. Murtha Neuroscience and Pain Institute, Johnstown, PA and the U.S. Dept. of Defense.
John Markman, MD is an independent contractor and on the speaker's bureau for Pfizer.

Disclosure of Discussion of non-FDA approved uses for pharmaceutical products and/or medical devices:
The University of Virginia School of Medicine, as an ACCME provider, requires that all faculty presenters identify and disclose any "off label" uses for pharmaceutical and medical device products. The University of Virginia School of Medicine recommends that each physician fully review all the available data on new products or procedures prior to instituting them with patients.

TO ENROLL

To enroll in the Medical Clinics of North America Continuing Medical Education program, call customer service at 1-800-654-2452 or visit us online at http://www.theclinics.com/home/cme. The CME program is available to subscribers for an additional fee of USD 205.

FORTHCOMING ISSUES

RECENT ISSUES

THE CLINICS ARE NOW AVAILABLE ONLINE!

Access your subscription at:
http://www.theclinics.com

GUEST EDITOR

HOWARD S. SMITH, MD, Director of Pain Management, Department of Anesthesiology, Albany Medical College, Albany, New York

CONTRIBUTORS

ALLEN CARL, MD, Professor, Department of Orthopaedic Surgery, Albany Medical Center, Albany, New York

GRACE CHANG, MD, MPH, Clinical Fellow, Massachusetts General Hospital Pain Center, Division of Pain Medicine, Department of Anesthesia and Critical Care, Massachusetts General Hospital, Harvard Medical School, Boston, Massachusetts

LUCY CHEN, MD, Instructor, Harvard Medical School, Massachusetts General Hospital Pain Center, Division of Pain Medicine, Department of Anesthesia and Critical Care, Massachusetts General Hospital, Harvard Medical School, Boston, Massachusetts

STEVEN P. COHEN, MD, Associate Professor, Pain Management Division, Department of Anesthesiology and Critical Care Medicine, Johns Hopkins School of Medicine; Department of Surgery, Walter Reed Army Medical Center, Washington, DC

ANTHONY DRAGOVICH, MD, Fellow in Pain Management, Anesthesia Service, Department of Surgery, Walter Reed Army Medical Center, Washington, DC

MOHAMMED A. KHALEEL, MS, Department of Orthopaedic Surgery, Albany Medical Center, Albany, NY

KENNETH L. KIRSH, PhD, Assistant Professor, Pharmacy Practice and Science, University of Kentucky, Lexington, Kentucky

ELIZABETH DEMERS LAVELLE, MD, Clinical Instructor, Department of Anesthesiology, Albany Medical Center, Albany, New York

LORI LAVELLE, DO, Medical Clinician, Department of Rheumatology, Altoona Arthritis and Osteoporosis Center, Altoona, Pennsylvania

WILLIAM LAVELLE, MD, Chief Resident, Department of Orthopaedic Surgery, Albany Medical Center, Albany, New York

JIANREN MAO, MD, PhD, Associate Professor, Harvard Medical School, Massachusetts General Hospital Pain Center, Division of Pain Medicine, Department of Anesthesia and Critical Care, Massachusetts General Hospital, Harvard Medical School, Boston, Massachusetts

JOHN D. MARKMAN, MD, Assistant Professor of Anesthesiology, Neurology, and Neurosurgery, University of Rochester School of Medicine and Dentistry, Rochester, New York; Director, The Pain Management Center at University of Rochester Medical Center, Rochester, New York

GARY McCLEANE, MD, FFARCSI, Consultant in Pain Management, Rampark Pain Centre, Lurgan, Northern Ireland, United Kingdom

ANNIE PHILIP, MD, Senior Instructor of Anesthesiology, University of Rochester School of Medicine and Dentistry, Rochester, New York

HOWARD S. SMITH, MD, Associate Professor of Anesthesiology, Director of Pain Management, Department of Anesthesiology, Albany Medical College, Albany, New York

CONTENTS

or even initial use, of opioids in pain patients. Therefore, it is essential that pain clinicians provide rationale for engaging in this modality of treatment and provide ample documentation in this regard. Thus, assessment and documentation are cornerstones for both protecting your practice and obtaining optimal patient outcomes while on opioid therapy. Several potential tools and documentation strategies are discussed that will aid clinicians in providing evidence for the continuation of this type of treatment for their patients.

Painful conditions of the musculoskeletal system, including myofascial pain syndrome, constitute some of the most important chronic problems encountered in a clinical practice. A myofascial trigger point is a hyperirritable spot, usually within a taut band of skeletal muscle, which is painful on compression and can give rise to characteristic referred pain, motor dysfunction, and autonomic phenomena. Trigger points may be relieved through noninvasive measures, such as spray and stretch, transcutaneous electrical stimulation, physical therapy, and massage. Invasive treatments for myofascial trigger points include injections with local anesthetics, corticosteroids, or botulism toxin or dry needling. The etiology, pathophysiology, and treatment of myofascial trigger points are addressed in this article.

Intra-articular injections are one method that physicians may use to treat joint pain. This method offers direct access to the source of pain for the troubled patient. Substances ranging from steroids to hyaluronic acid have been injected successfully into the various joints of the body in an attempt to provide relief for chronic joint pain. Anesthesiologists and orthopedic surgeons have begun to use intra-articular injections of local anesthetics for postoperative analgesia. The history, agents, and methods of intra-articular injections are reviewed.

Since the first use of intrathecal (IT) drug infusion systems in the early 1980s, these delivery systems have undergone numerous revisions making them more tolerable, easier to program, and longer lasting. Concurrent with technological advances, the indications for IT pump placement have also been continuously evolving, to the point where the most common indication is now noncancer pain. This article provides an evidence-based review of the indications, efficacy, and complications of IT drug therapy for the most commonly administered spinal analgesics.

This article reviews the evidence for several common interventional techniques for the treatment of chronic pain, including: intraspinal delivery of analgesics, reversible blockade with local anesthetics, augmentation with spinal cord stimulation, and ablation with radiofrequency energy or neurolytic agents. The role of these techniques is defined within the framework of a multidisciplinary approach to the neurobehavioral syndrome of chronic pain. Challenges to the study of the analgesic efficacy of procedural interventions are explored, as are the practical issues raised by their clinical implementation, with the aim of helping nonspecialist physicians identify the patients most likely to benefit from these approaches.

Back pain is a ubiquitous problem for developed countries. It is a source of disability for society and is a financial drain through lost wages and productivity. The treatment of spine-related pain has changed over the years; minimally invasive approaches are now favored. Despite this trend, surgeons still rely on decompressions of compressed neurologic structures and the fusion of painful motion segments. The history of treatments of spine-related pain as well as modern and minimally invasive techniques are reviewed.

Vertebral compression fractures occur more frequently than hip and ankle fractures combined. These fragility fractures frequently result in both acute and chronic pain, but more importantly are a source of increased morbidity and possibly mortality. Percutaneous veretebral augmentation offers a minimally invasive approach for the treatment of vertebral compression fractures. The history, technique, and results of vertebroplasty and kyphoplasty are reviewed. Both methods allow for the introduction of bone cement into the fracture site with clinical results indicating substantial pain relief in approximately 90% of patients.

ELSEVIER
SAUNDERS

Med Clin N Am 91 (2007) xi–xii

THE MEDICAL
CLINICS
OF NORTH AMERICA

Preface

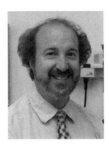

Howard S. Smith, MD
Guest Editor

Pain and suffering remain a significant dilemma. Pain continues to be among the most common reasons why patients seek medical attention (commonly for headache and back pain). Providing comfort and alleviation of pain and suffering remains a primary and crucial goal of patient care, as well as a great medical challenge. These issues of *Medical Clinics of North America, Pain Management* (Parts I and II), expose clinicians to a broad spectrum of available evaluation and management strategies.

The subjective nature of pain complaints, not uncommonly coupled with a lack of objective findings, continues to be troublesome for many clinicians who long for specific blood tests or imaging modalities that detect various pathophysiologies, in particular those which may help explain a patient's pain. Many physicians who are comfortable providing medical care to patients with hypertensive or diabetic issues do not have a similar level of comfort providing analgesia to patients with persistent noncancer pain.

In 2004, the American Society of Functional Neuroradiology (ASFNR) was founded to promote clinical applications of brain imaging techniques, such as magnetic resonance imaging (fMRI), positron emission tomography (PET), and an MRI method known as diffusion tensor imaging (DTI). It is hoped that these and other functional neuroradiologic techniques may eventually be clinically useful for patients suffering from pain and other symptoms.

In the Proceedings of the National Academy of Science (December 20, 2005), neuroscientists reported using fMRI to teach people with chronic

doi:10.1016/j.mcna.2007.01.007   *medical.theclinics.com*

pain to monitor and control their own brain activity (in specific regions)—
a high-tech version of biofeedback. Patients attempted to extinguish com-
puter-generated flames, and the intensity of the flames reflected MRI neural
activity in the patient's right anterior cingulated cortex (ACC)—a region
implicated in pain perception. Patients who were best at quelling the flames
(neural activity in the ACC), reported the most pain improvement after the
session.

Using genetics in the assessment of pain and its treatment has only just
begun. Waxman's group at Yale identified the first inherited painful neuropathy from a mutation producing a hyperpolarizing shift in activation and
depolarizing shift in steady-state activation. Studies of families with autoso-
mal dominant erythromelalgia (characterized by severe burning pain
in the limbs in response to mild thermal stimuli or moderate exercise) have
demonstrated mutations in SCN9A, the gene that encodes sodium channel
Na(v)1.7 and which is selectively expressed within nociceptive dorsal root
ganglion and sympathetic ganglion neurons. Other genetic analgesic treatment strategies may involve selectively dampening the expression of undesir-
able genes using RNA interference technologies. Future work may enable
viral rectors to deliver small interfering (siRNA) molecules to reduce or
eliminate mRNA with resultant long-term suppression of algesia-promoting
molecules.

It seems that the analgesic magic bullet is nonexistent, and the list of
analgesic targets continues to grow. Future clinical analgesic strategies
may include investigator-driven preclinical strategies, such as modulation
of bidirectional communications between neurons and glia, ablation or
inhibition of NK-1 expressing superficial dorsal horn cells, or intrathecal
cytokine therapy or proteosome-induced inhibition of ubiquitination
pathways.

Despite the explosion of preclinical research, the art of clinical pain medicine remains in its infancy. Optimally, individually designed mechanistic-
based targeted analgesic treatments can be tailored for specific patients,
thereby eliminating or reducing pain to minimal levels. Although clinicians
remain limited in their ability to identify specific cellular/molecular mechanisms contributing to an individual patient's pain complaints, it is our hope
that these volumes will help clinicians approach the evaluation and management of patients with persistent pain.

Howard S. Smith, MD
Albany Medical College
Department of Anesthesiology
47 New Scotland Avenue, MC-131
Albany, New York 12208

E-mail address: SmithH@mail.amc.edu

ELSEVIER
SAUNDERS

THE MEDICAL
CLINICS
OF NORTH AMERICA

Med Clin N Am 91 (2007) 177–197

Opioids for Persistent Noncancer Pain

Gary McCleane, MD, FFARCSI[a],*,
Howard S. Smith, MD, FACP[b]

[a]Rampark Pain Centre, 2 Rampark Dromore Road,
Lurgaqn BT66 7JH, Northern Ireland, UK
[b]Department of Anesthesiology, Albany Medical College,
47 New Scotland Avenue, MC 131 Albany, New York 12208, USA

No discussion of analgesia would be possible without mention of the opioid analgesics. These agents, both those classified as "mild" and "strong," are extensively used in the management of all types of pain—acute and chronic, neuropathic and nonneuropathic, that arising from cancer and that not arising from cancer—and their use is underpinned by extensive trial evidence and an abundance of practical experience. Indeed, an in-depth discussion of the pharmacologic and clinical aspects of opioid use could barely be served by a single journal issue, let alone a single article. Therefore, it would be simplistic to try to discuss the concept of opioid use in this article and hope that it would be in any way a comprehensive review. On the other hand, despite the 200 years that have passed since the chemical isolation of morphine, every year brings new understanding of the mode of action, propensity to cause side effects, and appropriate clinical use of opioids, and it is this "new" evidence as disclosed by recent publications on which this article concentrates.

Despite long experience with opioid use, prescribing habits are changing. Olsen and colleagues [1] have assessed the opioid use by American primary care physicians and found that opioids were prescribed in 5% of all visits between 1992 and 2001. The rate was 4.1% in 1992 through 1993 and rose to 6.3% in 1998 through 1999 with possession of Medicaid or Medicare and receiving a nonsteroidal anti-inflammatory drug (NSAID), increasing the chances of receiving an opioid while being of Hispanic origin, being in a health-maintenance organization, or living in the northeast or Midwest mitigating against opioid prescription. Undoubtedly with the increasing availability of modified strong opioid preparations, either in transdermal

---

* Corresponding author.
E-mail address: gary@mccleane.freeserve.co.uk (G. McCleane).

0025-7125/07/$ - see front matter © 2007 Elsevier Inc. All rights reserved.
doi:10.1016/j.mcna.2006.10.013   *medical.theclinics.com*

or oral formulations, and the increased advertising of their use by the pharmaceutical industry, there is an increased pressure to prescribe accompanied by an increased willingness to use opioids, particularly those that are classified as being strong (eg, clinically "pure" mu opioid agonists for severe pain).

With such use of strong opioids, particularly in the long term, questions of their effects with protracted use arise. At least some of the evidence is conflicting. Won and colleagues [2] report their findings of a study of 10,372 nursing home residents who had persistent pain. They found that 18.9% were taking short-acting opioids, whereas 3.3% were taking long-acting opioids. They found that there were no changes in cognitive status, mood status, or increased risk of depression with use of opioid analgesics. Furthermore, they found a decreased risk of falls with opioid use. In contrast, Vestergaard and colleagues [3] performed a nationwide survey of all patients sustaining a fracture in Denmark in 2000. This included 124,655 patients. Controls (373,962) were drawn from the background population. Morphine and other opiates were taken by 8.0% of the fracture subjects and by 3.2% of the control population. The odds ratio for sustaining a fracture were 1.47 with morphine, 2.23 with fentanyl, 1.39 with methadone, 1.36 with oxycodone, 1.54 with tramadol, 1.16 with codeine, and 0.86 with buprenorphine. Therefore, in this extensive review, the use of almost all opioids was association with an increased risk of fracture.

Aspects of the mode of action of opioids

A brief summary of the mode of action of opioids suggests that they achieve analgesia by interaction at four principle sites:

- Activating opioid receptors in the midbrain and turning on the descending inhibitory systems
- Activating opioid receptors on the second order pain transmission cells to prevent the ascending transmission of the pain signal
- Activating opioid receptors at the central terminals of C-fibers in the spinal cord
- Activating opioid receptors in the periphery to inhibit the activation of the nociceptors as well as inhibit cells that may release inflammatory mediators

The now well-known opioid receptors (mu, delta, and kappa) belong to the G-protein coupled receptor family. Agonist binding causes conformational changes that result in intracellular protein activation and inhibition of the activity of adenylyl cyclase. Adenylyl cyclase exists in 10 known forms. Kim and colleagues [4] have shown that, at least in mice, it is the adenylyl cyclase type 5 that is crucial in the analgesic and other effects of opioids. Specifically, they have shown that in mice that have genetic adenylyl cyclase type 5 absence, the behavioral effects of selective mu and delta opi-oid receptor agonists are lost, whereas the effects of selective kappa agonists are unaffected.

Under resting conditions, adenylate cyclase converts ATP into cyclic aden-osine monophosphate (cAMP). cAMP acts as a second messenger within the cell resulting in several events including the activation of protein kinases and gene transcription proteins. This induced-decrease in cAMP indirectly results in the inhibition of voltage-dependent calcium channels on presynaptic neu-rons, which are important in the release of neurotransmitter and transduction of neuronal communication (Fig. 1). Opioid receptors located on the presyn-aptic terminals of the nociceptive C-fibers and Aδ-fibers, when activated by an opioid agonist, will indirectly inhibit these voltage-dependent calcium channels by way of decreasing cAMP levels hence blocking the release of pain neurotransmitters such as glutamate, substance P, and calcitonin gene–related peptide from the nociceptive fibers resulting in analgesia.

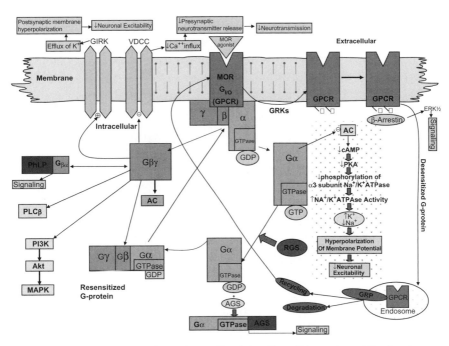

Fig. 1. Acute morphine (MOR) agonist-mediated signaling. *Abbreviations:* AC, adenylate cy-clase; AGS, activators of G-protein signaling; ERK ½, extra-cellular signal regulated kinase ½; GIRK, G-protein-activated inwardly rectifying potassium [K+] channels; GPCR, G-protein cou-pled receptor; GRKs, G-protein-coupled receptor kinases; GRP, G-protein-coupled phospha-tase; GTP, Guanine Triphosphate; MAPK, Mitogen-activated protein kinase; PhLP, Phosducin-like protein; PI3K, phosphatidyl inositol-3-kinase; PKA, protein kinase A; PLC, phos-pholipase C; VDCC, voltage-dependent calcium channels. (*From* Smith HS. Mechanism and modulation of Mu-opioid receptor agonist signaling. Journal of Cancer Pain and Symptom Pal-liation 2006;1:3–13; reprinted with permission from The Haworth Press, Inc. © Copyright 2006.)

Unfortunately our understanding of the multitude of effects induced by opioid administration is clouded by the presence of species variations. Berger and colleagues [5] have compared the presynaptic opioid receptors on noradrenergic and serotinergic neurons in human and rat neocortex. They have shown that in rats, mu opioid receptors modulate noradrenaline release, but 5HT release is only weakly affected by mu and kappa opioids. In contrast, noradrenaline release in human neocortex is modulated by way of delta opioid receptors, but 5HT release mainly by way of kappa opioid receptors.

It is now clear that opioids exert an influence in many areas of the central nervous system either to inhibit or influence nociceptive impulses or to adapt the physiologic responses to them. It may be possible that differing opioid receptors in particular areas of the central nervous system exert a differential influence on pain or the symptoms and signs exhibited along with pain. For example, Wang and colleagues [6] have examined the role of different types of opioid receptors in the thalamic nucleus submedius on allodynia in rats that have a spinal nerve ligation. They showed that this particular brain area is involved in the antiallodynic effect of opioids and that this action is mediated by mu-opioid but not delta- and kappa-opioid receptors in this neuropathic pain model.

Clinical effects of opioids

The last few years have seen the publication of several systematic reviews concerning various aspects of the effects of opioids. To a large extent these offer no surprises, but rather reassure that the widespread use of opioids in clinical practice is based on hard scientific evidence (Table 1).

What is lacking is any firm indication that any particular opioid has demonstrable superiority to others, and one is therefore left to select an opioid for clinical use based on personal experience and familiarity of the various drugs and their formulations in different clinical circumstances.

This has lead to more accepting attitudes from mainstream American medicine regarding the use of opioids for persistent noncancer pain [7]. However, the "opioid controversy" continues to the present. Portenoy [8] has illustrated various "opiophobic" versus "opiophilic" views in his comments predicting responses of American physicians to the recommendation for the appropriate use of opioids published by the UK Pain Society and Royal Colleges of Anaesthetists, General Practitioners, and Psychiatrists [9]. Kalso and colleagues [10] and Trescot and colleagues [11] have also published recommendations for using opioids in chronic noncancer pain.

Practicing in the "middle of the road" by employing the appropriate use of opioids in the context of good medical practice, as well as appropriate attention to the risk assessment and management of opioid abuse (ie, being cognizant of potential abuse, addiction, and diversion), has become known as "balance" [12–14].

Issues that surround the initiation (or maintenance) phase of Long-Term Opioid Therapy (LTOT) for Persistent Noncancer Pain (PNCP) include the use of: opioid "contracts" or agreements, goal-directed therapy agreements [15], a substance abuse history or "screening tool" for substance misuse, urine testing, unscheduled pill counts, and optimally some form of psychologic assessment (which could be an assessment by the provider), documentation tools (see article by Kirsh) as well as some sense of the "doctor–patient" relationship. Each clinic/clinician may use different items/tools in the practice—and there currently are no requirements to what some authors have referred to *as risk management plans.*

Perhaps one of the most important principles as a clinician in initiating and maintaining LTOT for PNCP is to "know where you are and where you are going." Goal-directed therapy agreements (GDTA) may be helpful when initiating LTOT for PNCP [15]. Clinicians are sometimes faced with patients in whom opioids were started or exculpated in efforts to achieve analgesia without clearly defined endpoints. This may yield patients remaining with severe pain on high-dose opioids. In efforts to clarify patient and clinician expectations and attempt to make expected treatment outcomes more finite and concrete, the use of some form of GDTAs may possess potential utility. As with opioid treatment agreements, GDTAs are not necessarily advocated for all patients or all practices, but merely suggested in situations in which clinicians deem them appropriate to use.

GDTAs should be tailored to each individual patient, clear and concise, reasonable for the patient to attain over a finite period of time, and optimally agreed upon by both patient and clinician. Examples may include increasing daily ambulation by a defined amount, increasing social/recreational activities by a defined amount, and so forth. By using GDTAs before instituting opioid therapy, clinicians can set defined criteria that need to be met to continue opioid therapy. In this manner, patients may be expected to reach certain reasonably attainable functional goals (which may need to be documented by their physical or behavioral therapist) to continue opioid therapy. The defined goals should be clearly stated in the GDTA. It seems optimal to institute the GDTA before instituting opioid therapy. The GDTA is essentially felt to be a "contractually" agreed upon realistic target of translational analgesia [15], which should be realized to continue therapy as is.

Although before LTOT there may not be any specific need for psychologic/psychiatric evaluations or psychologic testing, it seems prudent that clinicians should "know" a patient, and have an established provider–patient relationship before initiating LTOT for PNCP. Wasan and colleagues [16] reported that high levels of psychopathology (comprised mainly of depression, anxiety, and high neuroticism) are associated with diminished opioid analgesia in patients who have discogenic low back pain.

Eisenberg and colleagues [17] published a systematic review and metanalysis of trials evaluating the safety and efficacy of opioid agonists in the treatment of neuropathic pain of nonmalignant origin. Eisenberg and colleagues

MCCLEANE & SMITH

Table 1
Recent systematic reviews concerning opioid use (published in 2004–2006)

Clinical scenario	No. of trials analyzed	No. of patients	Outcomes
NSAIDs +/− opioids in cancer pain [60, 61]	42	3084	NSAID + opioid: no difference (4 of 14 papers); statistically insignificant benefit (1 of 14 papers); slight but statistically significant benefit (9 of 14 papers)
Oxycodone for cancer pain [62]	4	—*	Efficacy and tolerability of oxycodone similar to morphine
Oral transmucosal fentanyl for breakthrough pain in cancer [63]	4	393	Effective for cancer breakthrough pain
Efficacy of epidural	31	1343	72% of patients obtain "excellent" pain relief
Subarachnoid	28	722	62% of patients obtain "excellent" pain relief
Intracerebroventricular opioids in pain due to cancer [64]	13	337	73% of patients obtain "excellent" pain relief
Long-term oral opioid for chronic non-cancer pain [65]	16	1427	None of the studies were of good quality Insufficient evidence to produce conclusion
Opioids for chronic noncancer Pain [66]	41	6019	Weak and strong opioids outperform placebo for all types of chronic noncancer pain
Tramadol for neuropathic pain [67]	5	161	NNT of tramadol compared to placebo 3.5; NNH of tramadol compared to placebo 7.7
Opioids for noncancer pain [18]	15	1145	Short-term efficacy of opioids are good for bothneuropathic and musculoskeletal pain; 80% of patients experienced at least one adverse-event with opioid use; only 44% of 388 patients on open label treatment were still taking the opioid between 7 and 24 months after commencement

			Comments
Analgesia in postherpetic neuralgia [68]	31	—*	Strong opioids and tramadol effective, codeine ineffective
Opioids in neuropathic pain treatment [17]	22	—*	Opioids show effectiveness, high incidence of adverse effects
Mu agonists in treatment of evoked neuropathic pain [69]	9	—*	Dynamic allodynia significantly reduced; no consistent effect on static allodynia; -small number of studies hinders interpretation
NSAIDs and opioids for renal colic [70]	20	1613	NSAIDs more effective than opioids in reducing pain; higher incidence of adverse events with opioids compared to NSAIDs
Intra-articular morphine after knee arthroscopy [71]	46	—*	Few well-controlled studies; no added analgesic effect of intra-articular morphine compared to saline
Opioid switching [72]	—	—*	Opioid switching results in improvement in more than 50% of patients who have chronic pain with poor response to one opioid
Opioid side effects in chronic nonmalignant pain [73]	34	5546	Dry mouth 25% of patients; nausea 21%; constipation 15%; 22% withdraw from opioid therapy because of side effects

Abbreviations: NNH, numbers needed to harm; NNT, numbers needed to treat.
* Number of patients not indicated in review paper.

examined 22 studies that met inclusion criteria and were classified as short term (less than 24 hours; n = 14) or intermediate term (median = 28 days; range = 8–56 days; n = 8) trials. They reported that the short-term trials had contradictory results. However, all 8 intermediate-term trials demonstrated opioid efficacy for spontaneous neuropathic pain. A fixed-effects model meta-analysis of 6 intermediate-term trials showed mean posttreatment visual analog scale scores of pain intensity after opioids to be 14 units lower on a scale from 0 to 100 than after placebo (95% confidence interval -18 to -10; $P < .001$). As the mean initial pain intensity recorded from 4 of the intermediate-term trials ranged from 46 to 69, this 14-point difference was considered to correspond to a 20% to 30% greater reduction with opioids than with placebo.

Kalso and colleagues [18] analyzed data from 1145 patients initially randomized in 15 placebo-controlled trials of potent opioids used in the treatment of severe pain for efficacy and safety in chronic noncancer pain. Four studies tested intravenous opioids in neuropathic pain in a crossover design with 115 of 120 patients completing the protocols. Using either pain intensity difference or pain relief as the endpoint, all 4 intravenous studies reported average pain relief of 30% to 60% with opioid. Eleven studies (1025 patients) compared oral opioids with placebo for 4 days to 8 weeks. Six of the 15 trials that were included had an open-label follow-up of 6 to 24 months. The mean decrease in pain intensity in most studies was at least 30% with opioids and was comparable in neuropathic and musculoskeletal pain. Approximately 80% of patients noted at least one adverse effect. The most common adverse effects were constipation (41%), nausea (32%), and somnolence (29%). Only 44% of 388 patients on open-label treatments were still on opioids after therapy for between 7 and 24 months. Adverse effects and lack of efficacy were two common reasons for discontinuation.

Watson and colleagues [19] surveyed 102 patients who had PNCP in a neurologic practice followed by a neurologist every 3 months for 1 year or more (median 8 years, range 1–22 years). They reported that approximately one third of patients (34 out of 102) had a change in their pain status from either severe to moderate pain, as measured by a 0 to 10 numerical rating scale (mild = 1–3, moderate = 4–7, severe = 8–10); by category scale (absent, mild, moderate, severe, very severe); and by considering pain with movement. They queried patients as to whether they were satisfied with pain relief despite adverse events. Forty-five patients (44%) answered that they were satisfied and 57 (56%) replied that they were not satisfied. However, of the 86 patients assessed for disability, 47 (54%) had significant improvement in their disability status on opioids. Also, there was some pain improvement on opioids in 78 (91%) of 102 patients, and the patients chose to continue opioid therapy for some analgesia despite adverse effects.

Intraspinal drug infusion is an available option that may be used for the treatment of intractable persistent pain that is unresponsive to less-invasive approaches. In efforts to review current literature, revise the algorithm for drug selection developed in 2000, and develop current guidelines among other goals, the Polyanalgesic Consensus Conference 2003 was organized. Opioids have been and continue to be a mainstay agent for intraspinal therapy. In fact, the guidelines developed at the Polyanalgesic Consensus Conference 2003 suggest that the first-line intraspinal agent should be an opioid alone such as morphine sulfate or hydromorphone (and switch from one agent to another if the maximum dose is reached or side effects occur) [20].

Overall, the use of LTOT for PNCP may provide significant analgesia patients with minimal side effects for many years, however, it must be kept in mind that:

- LTOT may not be optimal for all patients.
- LTOT does not provide good or excellent analgesia in all patients.
- LTOT is not devoid of side effects.
- LTOT should be monitored in an effort to assess efficacy, side effects, and aberrant drug behavior.
- LTOT can be successfully withdrawn in selected patients who may do better without opioids.
- Prescribing LTOT for PNCP remains very much an art that may be used alone or in conjunction with other therapeutic options but typically not as a first-line agent for patients who have not tried previous treatments.

Analgesic tolerance

Definitions

The American Academy of Pain Medicine, the American Pain Society, and the American Society of Addiction Medicine recognize the following concensus definitions:

Addiction

Addiction is a primary, chronic, neurobiologic disease with genetic, psychosocial, and environmental factors influencing its development and manifestations. It is characterized by behaviors that include one or more of the following: impaired control over drug use, compulsive use, continued use despite harm, and craving.

Physical dependence

Physical dependence is a state of adaptation that is manifested by a drug class specific withdrawal syndrome that can be produced by abrupt cessation, rapid dose reduction, decreasing blood level of the drug, or administration of an antagonist.

Tolerance

Tolerance is a state of adaptation in which exposure to a drug indices changes that result in a diminuation of one or more of the drug's effects over time.

Perhaps the major impediment to more widespread acceptance of the concept of the use of strong opioids in chronic noncancer pain is the real chance of at some point needing to increase the dose of the opioid to achieve the same level of pain relief. It was not so long ago that we supposed in cancer pain management that increasing dose was required because the nociceptive stimulus increased with more widespread distribution of tumor as time progressed. An understanding of the interaction of opioids with various central nervous systems now shows that supposition to be simplistic.

Cholecystokinin

Cholecystokinin (CCK) is a peptide, originally thought to be confined to the gastrointestinal tract, but is now known to be corepresented in the CNS as well. CCK acts as an antiopioid peptide in that when it is administered along with an opioid analgesic in various animal pain models, the antinociceptive effect of the opioid is obtunded. If a CCK antagonist is administered, then the antinociceptive effect of the opioid is enhanced. Repeated administration of opioid increases the release of CCK and mirrors the decreasing effect of that repeatedly administered opioid. When established antinociceptive tolerance is found, it can be reversed by the administration of a CCK antagonist. When the CCK antagonist is administered from commencement of the opioid, antinociceptive tolerance is prevented [21,22].

Calcium/calmodulin-dependent protein kinase II

When mice are treated with morphine, tolerance develops as quickly as 2 to 6 hours. If the calcium/calmodulin-dependent protein kinase II inhibitor KN93 is administered to mice that have become tolerant to morphine, their sensitivity to morphine returns, suggesting that calcium/calmodulin-dependent protein kinase II has a direct effect on the development of opioid antinociceptive tolerance [23].

N-methyl-D-Aspartate

It is thought that the nucleus accumbens, part of the amygdala, plays an important part in drug abuse and dependence. When morphine is chronically administered to rats, the levels of the NR1 and NR2B subunits of the *N*-methyl-D-aspartate (NMDA) receptors in this region are significantly increased [24]. Not only do changes in NMDA receptor function occur in the brain, but also in the spinal dorsal horn chronic morphine exposure is associated with an enhanced NMDA receptor function, as measured electrophysiologically, and this again may be implicated in antinociceptive tolerance [25].

Glutamate

When morphine-tolerant mice are examined, they have significantly elevated levels of the vesicular glutamate transporter 1 and the synaptic vesicle-specific small G-protein Rab3A and that these elevated levels are associated with enhances spinal cord excitatory synaptic transmission, which in turn suppresses morphine-induced antinociception [26].

Calcium channel currents

In mice treated repeatedly with morphine and made tolerant to its effects, the effectiveness of mu opioid agonists to inhibit the normal calcium channel current in mu opioid receptors on sensory neurons is lost and has been postulated to have at least some part to play in opioid antinociceptive tolerance [27].

Gamma amino butyric acid

Gamma amino butyric acid (GABA) A receptor–mediated synaptic transmission is important in nociceptive processing and is a major target when opioids are administered. In the nucleus raphe magnus, a critical site for opioid analgesia, the GABA A receptor–mediated inhibitory postsynaptic current is significantly increased in morphine-tolerant animals. Protein kinase A inhibitors reverse this chronic morphine-induced synaptic adaptation of GABA-mediated inhibitory postsynaptic currents suggesting that chronic morphine exposure increases GABA synaptic activity [28].

Enkephalins

Mice that have genetic absence of preproenkephalin display blunted morphine antinociceptive tolerance but have normal conditioned place preference [29].

The above gives some examples of work recently published on analgesic tolerance with opioids. It makes it clear that analgesic tolerance with opioid use is multifactorial and so it may be naive to think that any one pharmacologic intervention could ever have a chance of preventing the onset of this troublesome side effect of opioid use.

Opioid side effects

Opioid-induced hyperalgesia

Although it is accepted that opioids are a most important treatment for pain, and in particular severe pain, there may be occasions in which it can induce hyperalgesia rather than pain relief [30,31]. This is most easily seen in humans when ultrashort-acting opioids are used. For example,

Angst and colleagues [32] have shown that the area of skin with induced mechanical hyperalgesia is significantly increased after discontinuation of a remifentanil infusion. They go on to shown that coadministration of the NMDA receptor antagonist S-ketamine along with remifentanil abolishes the enlargement of hyperalgesic skin seen when remifentanil is used alone. Similarly, Hood and colleagues [33] induced hyperalgesia by applying capsaicin to skin. Remifentanil infusions were commenced and run for 60 to 100 minutes. This remifentanil reduced the area of hyperalgesia. When the remifentanil was discontinued, areas of hyperalgesia and allodynia increased above pretreatment levels by approximately 180%.

Endocrine consequences of long-term administration of opioids

Abs and colleagues [34] have examined the endocrine consequences of long-term intrathecal opioid administration. Their subjects had a mean duration of opioid therapy of 27 months. Decreased libido and impotence were present in 23 of the 24 male subjects studied. Serum testosterone and free androgen were markedly lowered in treated as compared with control male subjects. Decreased libido was found in 22 of 32 women on long-term opioid therapy. All 21 premenopausal females developed either amenorrhea or an irregular menstrual cycle with ovulation in only 1 subject. Serum leutenising hormone, estradiol, and progesterone levels were all significantly lower in the opioid treatment subjects. When all subjects were considered together, the urinary-free cortisol excretion over 24 hours was significantly lower than in control subjects. Therefore, the large majority of men and women treated with long-term intrathecal opioid therapy developed hypogonadotrophic hypogonadism.

One option to address this problem in men is the use of a testosterone patch. Daniell and colleagues [35] report an open-label trial of the use of this patch in men who have opioid-induced androgen deficiency and found that use of a testosterone patch normalized hormone levels and seemed to improve several quality of life parameters, including sexual function.

Opioids and the immune system

It is becoming increasingly clear that opioid treatment can have effects on immune function. Morphine can decrease the effectiveness of several functions of both natural and adaptive immunity and significantly reduces cellular immunity. In contrast, buprenorphine has not affected cellular immune responses [36].

Constipation

Constipation is a predictable but troubling effect associated with opioid use. Ackerman and colleagues [37] have examined the rate of constipation in patients who have chronic pain receiving transdermal fentanyl and controlled release oxycodone. They included 877 patients using transdermal fentanyl and 1218 patients using controlled release oxycodone for at least 3 consecutive months in their analysis. Of these patients, 75 were judged to have constipation (28 transdermal fentanyl, 47 controlled release oxycodone). In patients over the age of 65, those taking oxycodone were judged to be 7.33 times more likely to be constipated than those using transdermal fentanyl.

Aspects of the use of individual opioids

Transdermal buprenorphine

Buprenorphine is increasingly being used in the management of pain, both related and unrelated to cancer. It seems to have marked antihyperalgesic effects, which increase its utility in the treatment of neuropathic pain. Sittl [38] suggests that the conventional conversion ratio of morphine to transdermal buprenorphine of 75:1 is questionable and should be changed to 100:1.

Transdermal fentanyl

Fentanyl is a synthetic phenylpiperidine mu opioid receptor agonist. It is approximately 80 times more potent than morphine, is highly lipophilic, and binds avidly to plasma proteins. After intramuscular administration of fentanyl citrate, the analgesic onset time is approximately 7 to 15 minutes; the time to peak analgesia may be extremely variable but could be approximated by 15 to 45 minutes, the analgesic duration is approximately 1 to 2 hours, and the elimination half-life is approximately 2 to 4 hours [39]. Fentanyl is largely metabolized by piperidine N-dealkylation to norfentanyl by way of hepatic microsomal CYP3A4 [39]. Amide hydrolysis to desproprionyl fentanyl and alkyl hydroxylation to hydroxyfentanyl are minor pathways [39]. Hydroxynorfentanyl is a minor secondary metabolite arising from N-dealkylation of hydroxyfentanyl [39].

Use of NSAIDs or weak opioids is the norm in the treatment of osteoarthritis pain. Even with such treatment, some patients continue to suffer pain. Langford and colleagues [40] report their study of 596 patients with defined osteoarthritis of the hip or knee who were randomized to receive either transdermal fentanyl or placebo. If taking NSAIDs before inclusion, they were permitted to continue them. Acetaminophen was offered as a rescue analgesic. Only 50% of patients completed the study. Transdermal fentanyl was shown to have a statistically significant pain-reducing effect than placebo. That said, reduction of visual analog scores (0–100) were 20 in the transdermal fentanyl group as opposed to 14.6 in the placebo group, giving a greater reduction with transdermal fentanyl of only 5.4 on this visual analog scale measurement. They also report that nausea, vomiting, and somnolence were more frequently encountered in the transdermal fentanyl group.

Oral transmucosal fentanyl citrate is a candied matrix formulation administered orally as a palatable lozenge on a stick. It is applied against the buccal mucosa; as it dissolves in saliva, a portion of the drug diffuses across the oral mucosa with the rest being swallowed and partially absorbed in the stomach and intestine. The bioavailability is approximately 50%. Oral transmucosal fentanyl citrate seems to be particularly well-suited for breakthrough pain (which is present in approximately two thirds of patients who have cancer with pain) because of its rapid onset. Meaningful analgesia may occur between 5 and 10 minutes after initiating oral transmucosal fentanyl citrate use. Peak plasma concentrations are achieved at 20 minutes and the duration of analgesia is approximately 2 hours [41]. The US Food and Drug Administration (FDA) issued an approvable letter for a Fentanyl buccal tablet in June 2006. Fentanyl effervescent buccal tablets enhance buccal delivery of fentanyl using a proprietary drug absorption system [42,43].

Oxycodone

In vitro experiments suggest that circulating metabolites of oxycodone are opioid receptor agonists. In a study of oxycodone in healthy human volunteers, Lalovic and colleagues [44] have shown that urinary metabolites of oxycodone derived from *N*-demethylation, noroxycodone, noroxymorphone, and alpha- and beta-noroxycodone account for approximately 45% of the total, whereas those products of *O*-demethylation, oxymorphone, and alpha- and beta-oxymorphol, and those of 6-keto-reduction, alpha- and beta-oxycodol account for 11% and 8%, respectively. Noroxycodone and noroxymorphone are the major metabolites in the circulation with elimination half-lives longer than that of oxycodone, but the uptake into the rat brain is significantly lower when compared with oxycodone. They conclude that the opioid effects of oxycodone are related to the parent drug and not to its metabolites.

One major question that continues to be of major relevance is whether individual opioids have distinct advantages over other members of this class. Staahl and colleagues [45] have compared the effects of morphine and oxycodone in healthy human volunteers. They used a crossover study design, so each subject received morphine and an equianalgesic dose of oxycodone. They have shown that both oxycodone and morphine are equipotent in pain modulation of induced skin and muscle pain. In contrast, when used for mechanically and thermally induced visceral pain of the esophagus, oxycodone produced significantly superior analgesia.

Marshall and colleagues [46] have assessed the cost of producing pain relief in patients who have osteoarthritis of the hip or knee when controlled release oxycodone or a combination of acetaminophen and oxycodone are used. They found that 62% of patients using controlled release oxycodone alone had pain relief as compared with 46% taking the combination of that drug and acetaminophen. Consequently, from an economic perspective, use of controlled release oxycodone alone was more cost-effective than use of the combination product.

Morphine

Codeine is to an extent metabolically converted to hydrocodone, but to date it has not been accepted that morphine is converted to hydromorphone. Cone and colleagues [47] report their study of 13 pain patients taking morphine at a high dose on a long-term basis and known not to be taking hydromorphone. Urine was collected and analysis revealed the presence of hydromorphone at low levels in 10 of the 13 subjects. This finding is of importance if urinary screening is undertaken in patients taking morphine to determine if they are abusing other opioids at the same time. If hydromorphone is found at low levels, it may be present because of metabolism of morphine and may not be an indication of concomitant hydromorphone use. If, however, the hydromorphone is found at high levels, then this is unlikely to be due solely to metabolism of morphine.

Codeine

Opioids are not used exclusively for the treatment of pain. Codeine, for example, has long been used as an antitussive. Smith and colleagues [48] report the results of their study of 21 patients who had chronic obstructive pulmonary disease and who were complaining of cough. These patients were given both codeine and placebo at differing times. They found that codeine was no more effective at reducing cough in patients who had long-standing pulmonary disease.

Remifentanil

The multifactorial nature of opioid analgesic tolerance has already been alluded to. Although antinociceptive tolerance to the effects of opioids is a well-defined entity in animal experimentation, its relevance to human clinical practice is still open to debate. In an interesting insight into analgesic tolerance with remifentanil, (an esterase-metabolized 4-anilidopiperidine ultra-short acting mu opioid receptor agonist with a half-life of approximately 3–10 minutes), Crawford and colleagues [49] describe their study of pediatric patients undergoing scoliosis surgery. Patients received either a continuous intraoperative remifentanil infusion or intermittent bolus dosing with morphine. All patients received morphine as a postoperative analgesic using a patient-controlled analgesia device. Cumulative postoperative morphine consumption was significantly higher in the remifentanil group by a margin of 30%, suggesting that intravenous infusion of remifentanil was associated with the onset of acute analgesic tolerance.

Oxymorphone

Oxymorphone, a 3-0-demethylation metabolite of oxycodone, is a potent opioid that has a 3 to 5 times higher mu opioid receptor affinity than morphine [50]. Oxymorphone has been studied for postsurgical pain in an oral immediate-release formulation and seems to be effective [51]. It has also been studied as an oral extended-release formulation and it seems that oxymorphone may be effective for moderate to severe pain secondary to osteoarthritis [52]. In June 2006, the FDA approved oxymorphone hydrochloride tablets (5 mg, 10 mg), and oxymorphone hydrochloride extended-release tables (5 mg, 10 mg, 20 mg, 40mg). It also seems that oxymorphone extended-release may be equianalgesic to oxycodone controlled-release at half the milligram daily dosage (with comparable safety) [53,54] and may be more potent than morphine at equianalgesic doses [55]. Oxymorphone extended-release uses TIMERx (Penwest Pharmaceuticals Co., Danbury, Connecticut) delivery system [56] to provide pharmacokinetic characteristics consistent with 12-hour dosing [57]. Major metabolites of oxymorphone include 6-OH-oxymorphone-3-glucuronide. It seems that oxymorphone extended-release dose not affect CYP2C9 or CYP3A4 metabolic pathways [58]. Noroxymorphone demonstrated a 3 fold and 10 fold higher affinity for the mu opioid receptor than oxycodone and noroxycodone, respectively [59].

Summary

Opioids, weak (referred to as opioids for mild to moderate pain) and strong (referred to as opioids for moderately severe to severe pain), have a well-deserved place in the management of pain, regardless of its type or duration. Evidence that has recently been published does nothing but confirm the utility of this class of drug in pain management. That said, extensive clinical experience with the use of opioids along with further recently published evidence confirms that opioids are drugs with a definite risk of causing adverse events, and therefore strong consideration must be given before opioid prescription about whether the intended benefit of use of a particular opioid merits its use despite the potential side effects and whether coprescription of other pharmacologic agents could reduce the risk of adverse events. In acute and cancer pain management, the decisions are easy. Opioids are justifiably widely prescribed. The major issue is their use as a long-term therapy for chronic pain conditions. Undoubtedly in the past there was a fear of the use of strong opioids in the management of chronic pain conditions. Many of these fears were exaggerated. It could be argued that we have now reached a stage where too little thought is given to the use of strong opioids in chronic pain treatment. If they were the only agents available, then it would be reasonable for them to be used extensively. However, in many chronic pain conditions we have useful additions to our therapeutic armamentarium and so the need to select a strong opioid should be reduced. For example, there is a weight of evidence that strong opioids can reduce human neuropathic pain. We now have an increasing array of drugs with proven efficacy in this condition. Some of these have specific indications (eg, pregabalin, lidocaine patch, and duloxetine); others do not and yet a body of evidence supports their use and they may have a reduced propensity to cause side effects (eg, $5HT_3$ antagonists, cholecystokinin antagonists, various antiepileptic agents). It could therefore be argued that we should not use strong opioids as an "automatic" first-line treatment option for the management of chronic pain conditions but reserve them for those patients who fail to respond to other lower risk options and in whom a proper consideration is given to the long-term consequences of strong opioid use (however, they also should certainly not be withheld as a "last ditch effort.").

The other remarkable feature of the recently published evidence is that we are still amassing insight into how opioids achieve their pain-relieving effects. This understanding becomes more complex as time progresses and shows that the opioids are medications with complex and diverse central and peripheral nervous system effects. To a certain extent, this gives scientific validity for their use. On the other hand, such complex interactions must be associated with a propensity to cause a multitude of effects other than just analgesia (eg, tolerance, addiction, paradoxical pain, and so forth). Also, prospective long-term well-designed studies of various opioids should be undertaken in elucidating certain adverse effects (eg, opioid effects on sleep and sleep-disordered breathing [sleep apnea]). The opioids therefore represent a well-validated treatment for both acute and chronic pain, but the problems associated with their use dictate that we still need to be looking for more efficacious and safer drugs to treat our patients. It could be contended that both a "not strong opioid for chronic pain" and a "strong opioid for all with chronic pain" mentalities are both flawed. Strong opioids should be used only after appropriate consideration of their use is made and only after thought is given to possible alternatives.

References

[1] Olsen Y, Daumit GL, Ford DE. Opioid prescriptions by US primary care physicians from 1992 to 2001. J Pain 2006;7:225–35.
[2] Won A, Lapane KL, Vallow S, et al. Long-term effects of analgesics in a population of elderly nursing home residents with persistent non-malignant pain. J Gerontol A Biol Sci Med Sci 2006;61:165–9.
[3] Vestergaard P, Rejnmark L, Mosekilde L. Fracture risk associated with the use of morphine and opiates. J Intern Med 2006;260:76–87.
[4] Kim KS, Lee KW, Lee KW, et al. Adenylyl cyclase type 5 (AC5) is an essential mediator of morphine action. Proc Natl Acad Sci USA 2006;103:3908–13.
[5] Berger B, Rothmaier AK, Wedekind F, et al. Presynaptic opioid receptors on noradrenergic and serotonergic neurons in the human as compared to the rat neocortex. Br J Pharmacol 2006;148:795–806.

[6] Wang JY, Zhao M, Yuan YK, et al. The roles of different subtypes of opioid receptors in mediating the nucleus submedius opioid-evoked antiallodynia in a neuropathic pain model in rats. Neuroscience 2006;138:1319–27.

[7] Chou R, Clark E, Helfan M, et al. Comparative efficacy and safety of long-acting oral opioids for chronic non-cancer pain: a systematic review. J Pain Symptom Manage 2003;26: 1026–48.

[8] Portenoy RK. Appropriate use of opioids for persistent non-cancer pain. Lancet 2004;364: 739–40.

[9] A consensus statement prepared on behalf of the Pain Society, the Royal College of Aneasthetists, the Royal College of General Practitioners, and the Royal College of Psychiatrists. Recommendations for the appropriate use of opioids for persistent non-cancer pain, the Pain Society, London (March 2004). Available at: http://www.painsociety.org/pdf/opioids_doc_ 2004.pdf. Accessed August 9, 2004.

[10] Kalso E, Allan L, Dellemijn PL, et al. Recommendations for using opioids in chronic non-cancer pain. Eur J Pain 2003;7:381–6.

[11] Trescot AM, Boswell MV, Atluri SL, et al. Opioid guidelines in the management of chronic non-cancer pain. Pain Physician 2006;9:1–39.

[12] A joint statement from 21 health organizations and the Drug Enforcement Administration. Promoting pain relief and preventing abuse of pain medications: a critical balancing act. Available at: http://www.medsch.wisc.edu/painpolicy/Consensus2.pdf. Accessed August 4, 2004.

[13] World Health Organization. Achieving balance in national opioids control policy: guidelines for assessment. Available at: http://who.int/medicines.docs/pagespublications/ qualitysafetypub.html.

[14] Zacny J, Bigelow G, Compton P, et al. College on problems of drug dependence task force on prescription opioid non-medical use and abuse: position statement. Drug Alcohol Depend 2003;69:215–32.

[15] Smith HS. Goal-directed therapy agreements. Journal of Cancer Pain and Symptom Palliation 2005;1:11–3.

[16] Wasan AD, Davar G, Jamison R. The association between negative effect and opioid analgesia in patients with discogenic low back pain. Pain 2005;177:450–61.

[17] Eisenberg E, McNicol ED, Carr DB. Efficacy and safety of opioid agonists in the treatment of neuropathic pain of nonmalignant origin: systematic review and meta-analysis trials. JAMA 2005;293:3043–52.

[18] Kalso E, Edwards JE, Moore RA, et al. Opioids in chronic non-cancer pain: a systematic review of efficacy and safety. Pain 2004;112:372–80.

[19] Watson CP, Watt-Watson JH, Chipman ML. Chronic noncancer pain and the long term utility of opioids. Pain Res Manag 2004;9:19–24.

[20] Hassenbusch SJ, Portenoy RK, Cousins M, et al. Polyanalgesic Consensus Conference 2003: an update on the management of pain by intrapsinal drug delivery—report of an expert panel. J Pain Symptom Manage 2004;27:540–63.

[21] McCleane GJ. The role of cholecystokinin antagonists in human pain management: a review. Journal Neuropathic Pain Symptom Palliation 2005;2:37–44.

[22] McCleane GJ. Cholecystokinin antagonists: can they augment opioid-derived analgesia? Journal Opioid Management 2005;1:273–9.

[23] Tang L, Shukla PK, Wang LX, et al. Reversal of morphine antinociceptive tolerance and dependence by the acute supraspinal inhibition of Ca $(2 +)$/calmodulin-dependent protein kinase II. J Pharmacol Exp Ther 2006;317:901–9.

[24] Bajo M, Crawford EF, Roberto M, et al. Chronic morphine treatment alters expression of N-methyl-D-aspartate receptor subunits in the extended amygdala. J Neurosci Res 2006; 83:532–7.

[25] Zhao M, Joo DT. Subpopulation of dorsal horn neurons displays enhanced N-methyl-D-aspartate receptor function after chronic morphine exposure. Anesthesiology 2006;104:815–25.

[26] Suzuki M, Narita M, Narita M, et al. Chronic morphine treatment increases the expression of vesicular glutamate transporter 1 in the mouse spinal cord. Eur J Pharmacol 2006;535: 166–8.

[27] Johnson EE, Chieng B, Napier I, et al. Decreased mu-opioid receptor signaling and a reduction in calcium current density in sensory neurons from chronically morphine-treated mice. Br J Pharmacol 2006;148:947–55.

[28] Ma J, Pan ZZ. Contribution of brainstem GABA (A) synaptic transmission to morphine analgesic tolerance. Pain 2006;122:163–73.

[29] Marquez P, Baliram R, Gajawada N, et al. Differential involvement of enkephalins in analgesic tolerance, locomotor sensitization, and conditioned place preference induced by morphine. Behav Neurosci 2006;120:10–5.

[30] Mao J. Opioid-induced abnormal pain sensitivity. Curr Pain Headache Rep 2006;10: 67–70.

[31] Angst MS, Clarke JD. Opioid-induced hyperalgesia: a qualitative systematic review. Anesthesiology 2006;104:570–87.

[32] Angst MS, Koppert W, Pahl I, et al. Short-term infusion of the mu-opioid agonist remifentanil in humans causes hyperalgesia during withdrawal. Pain 2003;106:49–57.

[33] Hood DD, Curry R, Eisenach JC. Intravenous remifentanil produces withdrawal hyperalgesia in volunteers with capsaicin-induced hyperalgesia. Anesth Analg 2003;97:810–5.

[34] Abs R, Verhelst J, Maeyaert J, et al. Endocrine consequences of long-term intrathecal administration of opioids. J Clin Endocrinol Metab 2000;85:2215–22.

[35] Daniell HW, Lentz R, Mazer NA. Open-label pilot study of testosterone patch therapy in men with opioid-induced androgen deficiency. J Pain 2006;7:200–10.

[36] Sacerdote P. Opioids and the immune system. Palliat Med 2006;20S:S9–15.

[37] Ackerman SJ, Knight T, Schein J, et al. Risk of constipation in patients prescribed fentanyl transdermal system or oxycodone hydrochloride controlled-release in a California Medicaid population. Consult Pharm 2004;19:118–32.

[38] Sittl R. Transdermal buprenorphine in cancer pain and palliative care. Palliat Med 2006;20S: S25–30.

[39] Janicki PK, Parris WC. Clinical Pharmacology of opioids. In: Smith HS, editor. Drugs For Pain. Philadelphia: Hanley and Belfus; 2003. p. 97–118.

[40] Langford R, McKenna F, Ratcliffe S, et al. Transdermal fentanyl for improvement of pain and functioning in osteoarthritis: A randomized, placebo-controlled trial. Arthritis Rheum 2006;54:1829–37.

[41] Lichtor JL, Sevarino FB, Joshi GP, et al. The relative potency of oral transmucosal fentanyl citrate compared with intravenous morphine in the treatment of moderate to severe post-operative pain. Anesth Analg 1999;89:732–8.

[42] Pather SI, Siebert JM, Hontz J, et al. Enhanced buccal delivery of fantanyl using the OraVescent drug delivery system. Drug Deliv Tech 2001;1:54–7.

[43] Durfee S, Messina J, Khankari R. Fentanyl effervescent buccal tablets: enhanced buccal absorption. Am J Drug Deliv 2006;4:1–5.

[44] Lalovic B, Kharasch E, Hoffer C, et al. Pharmacokinetics and pharmacodynamics of oral oxycodone in healthy human subjects: role of circulating active metabolites. Clin Pharmacol Ther 2006;79:461–79.

[45] Staahl C, Christrup LL, Andersen SD, et al. A comparative study of oxycodone and morphine in a multi-modal, tissue-differentiated experimental pain model. Pain 2006;123:28–36.

[46] Marshall DA, Strauss ME, Pericak D, et al. Economic evaluation of controlled-release oxycodone vs oxycodone-acetaminophen for osteoarthritis pain of the hip or knee. Am J Manag Care 2006;12:205–14.

[47] Cone EJ, Heit HA, Caplan YH, et al. Evidence of morphine metabolism to hydromorphone in pain patients chronically treated with morphine. J Anal Toxicol 2006;30:1–5.

[48] Smith J, Owen E, Earis J, et al. Effect of codeine on objective measurement of cough in chronic obstructive pulmonary disease. J Allergy Clin Immunol 2006;117:831–5.

[49] Crawford MW, Hickey C, Zaarour C, et al. Development of acute opioid tolerance during infusion of remifentanil for pediatric scoliosis surgery. Anesth Analg 2006;102:1662–7.

[50] Childers SR, Creese I, Snowman AM, et al. Opiate receptor binding affected differentially by opiates and opioid pep tides. Eur J Pharmacol 1979;55:11–8.

[51] Gimbel J, Ahdieh H. The efficacy and safety of oral immediate release oxymorphone for postsurgical pain. Anesth Analg 2004;99:1472–7.

[52] Matsumoto AK, Babul N, Ahdieh H. Oxymorphone extended-release tablets relieve moderate to severe pain and improve physical function in osteoarthritis: results of a randomized double-blind, placebo—and active—controlled phase III trial. Pain Med 2005;6: 357–66.

[53] Gabrail NY, Dvergsten C, Ahdieh H. Establishing the dosage equivalency of oxymorphone extended release and oxycodone controlled release in patients with moderate to severe cancer pain. Curr Med Res Opin 2004;20:911–8.

[54] Hale ME, Dvergsten C. Gimbel. Efficacy and safety of oxymorphone extended release in chronic low back pain: results of a randomized, double-blind, placebo—and active-controlled phase III study. J Pain 2005;6:21–8.

[55] Sloan P, Slatkin N, Ahdieh H. Effectiveness and safety of oral extended-release oxymorphone for the treatment of cancer pain: a pilot study. Support Care Cancer 2005;13:57–65.

[56] Pharmaceuticals P. TIMERx control release delivery systems. Available at: http://www.penwest.com/timerx.html. Accessed January 10, 2005.

[57] Adams MP, Ahdieh H. Pharmacokinetics and does-proportionality of oxymorphone extended release and its metabolites: results of a randomized crossover study. Pharmacotherapy 2004;24:468–76.

[58] Adams MP, Ahdieh H. Single- and multiple-dose pharmacokinetic and dose-proportionality study of oxymorphone immediate-release tablets. Drugs R D 2005;6:91–9.

[59] Lalovic B, Phillips B, Risler LL, et al. Quantitative contribution of CYP2D6 and CYP3A to oxycodone metabolism in human liver and intestinal microsomes. Drug Metab Dispos 2004; 32:447–54.

[60] McNichol E, Strassels SA, Goudas L, et al. NSAIDs or paracetamol, alone or combined with opioids, for cancer pain. Cochrane Database Syst Rev 2005;1:CD005180.

[61] McNichol E, Strassels S, Goudas L, et al. Nonsteroidal anti-inflammatory drugs, alone or combined with opioids, for cancer pain: a systematic review. J Clin Oncol 2004;22: 1975–92.

[62] Reid CM, Martin RM, Sterne JA, et al. Oxycodone for cancer-related pain: meta-analysis of randomized controlled trials. Arch Intern Med 2006;166:837–43.

[63] Zeppetella G, Ribeiro MD. Opioids for the management of breakthrough (episodic) pain in cancer patients. Cochrane Database Syst Rev 2006;1:CD004311.

[64] Ballantyne JC, Carwood CM. Comparative efficacy of epidural, subarachnoid, and intracerebroventricular opioids in patients with pain due to cancer. Cochrane Database Syst Rev 2005;1:CD005178.

[65] Chou R, Clark E, Helfand M. Comparative efficacy and safety of long-acting oral opioids for chronic non-cancer pain: a systematic review. J Pain Symptom Manage 2004;28:194–5.

[66] Furlan AD, Sandoval JA, Mailis-Gagnon A, et al. Opioids for chronic noncancer pain: a meta-analysis of effectiveness and side effects. CMAJ 2006;174:1589–94.

[67] Duhmke RM, Cornblath DD, Hollingshead JR. Tramadol for neuropathic pain. Cochrane Database Syst Rev 2004;2:CD003726.

[68] Hempenstall K, Nurmikko TJ, Johnson RW, et al. Analgesic therapy in postherpetic neuralgia: a quantitative systematic review. PLoS Med 2005;2:164.

[69] Eisenberg E, McNichol ED, Carr DB. Efficacy of mu-opioid agonists in the treatment of evoked neuropathic pain: systematic review of randomized controlled trials. Eur J Pain 2006;10:667–76.

[70] Holdgate A, Pollock T. Systematic review of the relative efficacy of non-steroidal anti-inflammatory drugs and opioids in the treatment of acute renal colic. BMJ 2004;328:1401.

[71] Rosseland LA. No evidence for analgesic effect of intra-articular morphine after knee arthroscopy: a qualitative systematic review. Reg Anesth Pain Med 2005;30:83–98.

[72] Mercadante S, Bruera E. Opioid switching: a systematic and critical review. Cancer Treat Rev 2006;32:304–15.

[73] Moore RA, McQuay HJ. Prevalence of opioid adverse events in chronic non-malignant pain: systematic review of randomised trials of oral opioids. Arthritis Res Ther 2005;7:1046–51.

ELSEVIER
SAUNDERS

THE MEDICAL
CLINICS
OF NORTH AMERICA

Med Clin N Am 91 (2007) 199–211

Opioid Tolerance and Hyperalgesia

Grace Chang, MD, MPH, Lucy Chen, MD,
Jianren Mao, MD, PhD*

*Massachusetts General Hospital Pain Center, Division of Pain Medicine, Department
of Anesthesia and Critical Care, Massachusetts General Hospital, Harvard Medical
School, Boston, MA 02114, USA*

Opioids are well recognized as the analgesics of choice, in many cases, for treating severe acute and chronic pain. Exposure to opioids, however, can lead to two seemingly unrelated cellular processes, the development of opioid tolerance and the development of opioid-induced pain sensitivity (hyperalgesia). The converging effects of these two phenomena can significantly reduce opioid analgesic efficacy, as well as contribute to the challenges of opioid management. This article will review the definitions of opioid tolerance (particularly to the analgesic effects) and opioid-induced hyperalgesia, examine both the animal and human study evidence of these two phenomena, and discuss their clinical implications. The article will also differentiate the phenomena from other aspects related to opioid therapy, including physical dependence, addiction, pseudoaddiction, and abuse.

Opioid tolerance and opioid-induced hyperalgesia

Opioid tolerance is a phenomenon in which repeated exposure to an opioid results in decreased therapeutic effect of the drug or need for a higher dose to maintain the same effect [1]. There are several aspects of tolerance relevant to this issue [2]:

Innate tolerance is the genetically determined sensitivity, or lack thereof, to an opioid that is observed during the first administration. *Acquired tolerance* can be divided into pharmacodynamic, pharmacokinetic, and learned tolerance [3].

Pharmacodynamic tolerance refers to adaptive changes that occur within systems affected by the opioid, such as opioid-induced changes in receptor density or desensitization of opioid receptors, such that response to a given

---

* Corresponding author.
E-mail address: jmao@partners.org (J. Mao).

0025-7125/07/$ - see front matter © 2007 Elsevier Inc. All rights reserved.
doi:10.1016/j.mcna.2006.10.003   *medical.theclinics.com*

concentration of the drug is reduced. There is increasing evidence that many of the mechanisms related to this type of tolerance involve the N-methyl-D-aspartate (NMDA) receptor.

Pharmacokinetic tolerance refers to changes in the distribution or metabolism of the opioid after repeated drug administrations that result in reduced concentrations of the opioid in the blood or at the sites of drug action. The most common mechanism of this phenomenon is an increase in the rate of metabolism of the opioid.

Learned tolerance is a reduction in the effects of an opioid as a result of mechanisms that are learned. One type of learned tolerance is *conditioned* or *associative tolerance*, which is a learned mechanism that develops when environmental cues are consistently paired with the administration of the drug. When the opioid affects homeostasis by causing sedation or decreasing gut motility, there is a reflex counteraction or adaptation to restore homeostasis, which prevents the full manifestation of the drug's effect. If the opioid is taken under novel circumstances, its effects are enhanced and tolerance is reduced.

Despite the above classifications of opioid tolerance, the clinical utility of such classifications remain to be seen. However, understanding various aspects of opioid tolerance would be likely to aid the investigation into the mechanisms of opioid tolerance.

There have been many studies that have reported that opioid administration can unexpectedly cause hyperalgesia (enhanced pain response to noxious stimuli) and allodynia (pain elicited by innocuous stimuli). This phenomenon can be seen with both acute and chronic administration of opioids and high doses of opioids, and has been observed in both animals and humans. A review of the clinical experiences of more than 750 patients receiving epidural or spinal morphine over a mean period of 4 months showed that many patients developed hyperesthesia (increased sensitivity to sensory stimuli) and allodynia [4]. Studies have shown that the NMDA receptor is also involved in hyperalgesia, as well as other receptors and neuropeptides.

The relative contribution of opioid tolerance versus opioid-induced hyperalgesia to the overall clinical picture is not known from either animal or human studies. What has been known is that the effect of the combination of these two phenomena is seen as an apparent decrease in analgesic efficacy (*apparent opioid tolerance*). It is important for clinicians to be familiar with these two mechanisms so that a decrease in opioid analgesic efficacy is not automatically interpreted as opioid tolerance and treated with dose escalation. Rather, clinicians should consider that increased pain might be a result of opioid tolerance, opioid-induced hyperalgesia, or disease progression and manage the opioid regimen accordingly.

Evidence from animal studies for opioid antinociceptive tolerance

Many studies have demonstrated the development of tolerance in various animal species. The administration of opioids will evoke a dose-dependent increase in the latency of response to thermal, chemical, and mechanical nociceptors [5,6]. However, with repeated exposure, the effect produced by a given dose of opioid will decrease in magnitude or the duration of action of the opioid will decrease. In addition, studies using continuous opioid infusions by different routes have shown tolerance to be dose-dependent, time-dependent, and receptor-specific, as well as reversible [7,8].

Tolerance to the analgesic effect of opioids is best shown pharmacologically by a rightward displacement of the analgesic dose-effect curve. Studies in the 1970s showed that repeated daily systemic injections of morphine to mice or rats produced significant rightwards shifts in the antinociceptive effects of the opioid [9,10]. Repeated systemic or intrathecal injections of morphine also produced a rightward shift in dose-response curves for intrathecal morphine in the hot-plate and tail-flick tests [11]. Also, prolonged exposure to morphine pellets implanted subcutaneously produced a shift to the right in the dose-effect curves for test doses of morphine given either supraspinally or intrathecally [12].

Evidence from animal studies for opioid-induced hyperalgesia

Many studies using various animal models also have demonstrated opioid-induced hyperalgesia, either with systemic or spinal administration of opioids. Large doses of intrathecal morphine are associated with nonspecific hyperalgesic and hyperesthesic responses [13]. In another study, rats given large (50 μg) intrathecal bolus injections of morphine showed nonspecific pain-related behaviors such as biting and scratching at dermatomes corresponding to the injection site, and aggressive behaviors in response to light brushing of the flanks [14].

More recent studies [15] also show that repeated opioid administration, at a clinical relevant dose range, can lead to a progressive and lasting reduction of baseline nociceptive thresholds, resulting in an increase in pain sensitivity. Rats receiving repeated intrathecal morphine administration (10 or 20 μg) over a 7-day period show a progressive reduction of baseline nociceptive thresholds [16–18]. This reduction is also seen in animals after subcutaneous fentanyl boluses using the Randall-Sellitto test, in which a constantly increasing pressure is applied to a rat's hind paw [19,20]. The decreased baseline nociceptive thresholds lasted as long as 5 days after the cessation of four fentanyl bolus injections. A similar phenomenon has been observed in animals with repeated heroin administration [21].

Opioid-induced hyperalgesia has also been observed with opioid withdrawal. It is possible that decreased baseline nociceptive thresholds observed in animals treated with opioid boluses may reflect a subliminal withdrawal in which changes in baseline nociceptive thresholds might precede other withdrawal signs such as wet-dog shaking and jumping. In this regard, a progressive reduction of baseline nociceptive thresholds has also been demonstrated in animals receiving continuous intrathecal opioid infusion via osmotic pumps. Moreover, opioid-induced pain sensitivity including thermal hyperalgesia and tactile allodynia is observed in these animals even when an opioid infusion continues [16,22], suggesting the involvement of active cellular mechanisms in the process.

Evidence from human studies for opioid analgesic tolerance

There are case reports and studies [23] that provide evidence for the development of acute tolerance to the analgesic effects of opioids. A study of pediatric scoliosis surgery patients who were either given a continuous infusion of remifentanil or intermittent morphine intraoperatively showed that there was a 30% higher postoperative morphine requirement in patients who received continuous remifentanil, with no difference in pain and sedation scores [24]. Another study of abdominal surgery patients also showed that those patients receiving large-dose intraoperative remifentanil had significantly higher postoperative pain scores and morphine requirement [25].

The evidence for the development of tolerance to the analgesic effects of opioids with chronic administration has been mixed. Many of the studies were in cancer patients with severe pain and showed that they maintained a stable opioid dose (for weeks to years) even with different routes of administration [3,4,26]. Although it is generally agreed that tolerance to the analgesic properties of opioids occurs in patients with malignant pain, dose escalation is thought to be mostly a result of disease progression rather than the development of pharmacodynamic tolerance.

There have been fewer studies of patients with nonmalignant chronic pain. Although chronic pain patients have been observed to require escalating opioid doses to maintain adequate analgesia, several studies have not shown dose escalation and tolerance to be a significant problem. A study of intrathecal morphine in nonmalignant pain showed that dose escalation was related to worsening pathology [27]. Other retrospective studies, including one of patients in an orthopedic spine clinic, have also shown that opioid dosages remained stable over a period of 3 years [3,28]. Indeed, the controversy of development of tolerance to the analgesic effects of opioids with chronic administration may be the result of incorrectly using dose escalation as a measure of tolerance. This is because dose escalation can be affected by many other variables, including disease progression and coexisting psychological issues such as depression and anxiety. Recently, there was a preliminary prospective study in which six chronic low back pain patients were assessed for both opioid tolerance and opioid-induced hyperalgesia using quantitative sensory testing (cold and heat) before and after the institution of oral morphine therapy [29]. Preliminary results showed hyperalgesia and tolerance with cold but no hyperalgesia with heat or analgesic tolerance to heat pain.

Evidence in human studies for tolerance to opioid side effects

Side effects of opioids after initial administration include sedation, nausea, vomiting, respiratory depression, miosis, constipation, and euphoria/dysphoria. Studies have shown that tolerance to sedation, nausea, and respiratory depression can occur rapidly, while tolerance to constipation and miosis is minimal.

Tolerance to the sedative and cognitive effects of opioids can occur rapidly. Usually sedation and cognitive impairment occur at the start of treatment or after a dose increase. One study showed that patients had significant cognitive impairment after a dose increase while patients on a stable regimen had no impairment [30]. In addition, patients seemed to be less aware of cognitive impairment compared with other side effects. If patients continue to be impaired by sedation, one can consider changing the dosing regimen to smaller and more frequent administrations. Alternatively, one could also use oral methylphenidate or modafinil to reduce sedation, if the opioid dose escalation is considered to be necessary for pain management.

The incidence of nausea has been estimated to occur in 40% of patients, while vomiting has been estimated to occur in 15% of patients. These effects usually resolve in a few days and patients can be given antiemetics while they have these symptoms [3].

Respiratory depression is a significant side effect of opioid administration as all opioids can depress the respiratory center in the brainstem. Tolerance to this effect develops rapidly and especially with repeated dosing but it is important for clinicians to be aware of the potential for respiratory arrest, especially in opioid-naïve patients receiving large doses or certain opioids (eg, methadone) with different pharmacokinetic profiles.

Constipation is a common side effect of opioid treatment and one to which there is little development of tolerance. Since opioids bind directly to peripheral opioid receptors in the gastrointestinal tract, there is decreased peristalsis; decreased biliary, pancreatic, and intestinal secretions; and increased ileocecal and anal sphincter tone. This leads to increased stool transit time and dessication of feces. In severe cases, patients can get narcotic bowel syndrome, which consists of nausea and vomiting, stomach discomfort, constipation, abdominal distention, and colonic obstruction. For these reasons, patients should always be on an aggressive bowel regimen while undergoing opioid treatment.

Evidence from human studies for opioid-induced hyperalgesia

Unlike laboratory animal studies in which changes in baseline nociceptive thresholds are measured in a controlled setting, it is difficult to determine whether changes in pain levels occur clinically following opioid administration [15]. It is challenging to distinguish pharmacological tolerance from hyperalgesia when efficacy of analgesia is usually based on subjective pain scores. However, there is still some evidence that suggests that opioid-induced hyperalgesia may be present clinically.

As previously discussed, there have been reports and studies showing decreased analgesic efficacy after intraoperative remifentanil infusion [22–24]. It should be noted these observations do not adequately distinguish whether what appears on the surface to be the development of opioid tolerance is actually due to pharmacologic tolerance, opioid-induced hyperalgesia, or both. One indication for the presence of opioid-induced hyperalgesia is the observation that patients treated intraoperatively with remifentanil reported more postoperative pain than the matched nonopioid controls. The level of postoperative pain should be comparable between the two groups if there was only the development of pharmacologic tolerance without opioid-induced hyperalgesia.

Empirical observations have suggested that pain sensitivity differs between normal subjects and those with opioid addiction [31–33]. Recently it has been reported that pain sensitivity to experimental pain stimulation is increased in opioid addicts [34]. Furthermore, those former opioid addicts maintained on methadone reported additional enhancement of pain sensitivity as compared with matched former opioid addicts not on methadone maintenance, suggesting that a prolonged methadone maintenance program may further worsen abnormal pain sensitivity in former opioid addicts.

There have been many recent case reports of cancer patients with high-dose opioid-induced hyperalgesia whose pain resolved after reduction in dose [35–37]. This has also been observed in chronic nonmalignant pain patients [38]. However, except for one recent preliminary study (see Chu and colleagues [29]), there is lack of controlled clinical studies and such studies are urgently needed to further evaluate clinical approaches to differentiation and management of pharmacologic tolerance versus opioid-induced hyperalgesia.

Mechanisms mediating opioid-induced hyperalgesia and antinociceptive tolerance

Studies suggest that opioid-induced hyperalgesia and antinociceptive tolerance may have mechanisms in common with neuropathic pain after peripheral nerve injury [39]. Both are associated with greatly reduced analgesic effect of morphine and are sensitive to reversal by NMDA antagonists. Activation of NMDA receptors by glutamate causes sensitization of spinal neurons. NMDA receptor-mediated central sensitization has been associated with opioid-induced hyperalgesia and enhanced nociception in chronic pain states. Blockade and reversal of opioid tolerance by NMDA receptor antagonists have been observed, demonstrating the importance of the NMDA receptor in the development of tolerance. Studies have also shown that hyperalgesia caused by fentanyl or heroin, as well as naloxone-mediated opiate withdrawal, was also blocked by NMDA receptor antagonists.

Recent evidence (see Mao [15]) also suggests that prolonged exposure to opioids induces neuroplastic changes resulting in the enhanced ability of the neuropeptides cholecystokinin (CCK) to excite pathways arising from the rostroventromedial medulla (RVM). This mechanism enhances morphine-induced pain and tolerance and leads to an up-regulation of spinal dynorphin content. Pathologically elevated levels of dynorphin then promote the release of excitatory neurotransmitters, which is pronociceptive and clinically manifests as increased pain and is seen as antinociceptive tolerance.

Clinical implications of opioid-induced hyperalgesia and antinociceptive tolerance

A diminishing opioid analgesic efficacy during opioid treatment is often considered a sign of pharmacological tolerance, assuming there is no apparent disease progression. Escalation of opioid doses has been a common approach to improve analgesia. However, this conventional practice of dose escalation needs to be revisited in light of both animal and human study evidence of paradoxical opioid-induced hyperalgesia. Apparent opioid tolerance is not synonymous with pharmacological tolerance, which calls for an increase in opioid dose, but may be the first sign of opioid-induced hyperalgesia, suggesting, instead, a need for opioid dose reduction. The important issue is how to distinguish the elements of apparent opioid tolerance and consider the "differential diagnosis" [40] for increased pain in clinical settings.

There are two other main categories of factors that can contribute to declining analgesia, besides tolerance: increased activity in nociceptive pathways and psychological processes. Increased activity in nociceptive pathways can include (1) increasing activation of nociceptors in the periphery because of mechanical factors (tumor growth) biochemical changes (inflammation), or peripheral neuropathic processes (neuroma formation) and (2) increased activity in central nociceptive pathways because of central neuropathic processes (sensitization, shift in receptive fields, or change in modulatory processes).

Psychological processes can include increased psychological distress (anxiety or depression), change in the cognitive state leading to altered pain perception or reporting (delirium), and conditioned pain behavior that is independent of the drug. There are several issues related to opioid-induced hyperalgesia, as discussed in the following paragraphs.

Opioid-induced hyperalgesia versus preexisting pain

Several features of opioid-induced pain observed in animal and human studies would be helpful in making distinctions between opioid-induced and preexisting pain. First, since opioid-induced hyperalgesia would conceivably exacerbate a preexisting pain condition, pain intensity should be increased above the level of preexisting pain following opioid treatment in the absence of apparent disease progression. Second, opioid-induced hyperalgesia would be diffuse, less defined in quality, and beyond the distribution of a preexisting pain state, given that the underlying mechanisms of opioid-induced hyperalgesia involve neural circuits and extensive cellular and molecular changes. Third, quantitative sensory testing may reveal changes in pain threshold, tolerability, and distribution patterns associated with the development of hyperalgesia. These parameters may also help make distinctions between the exacerbation of preexisting pain and opioid-induced pain. Fourth, undertreatment of a preexisting pain or the development of pharmacologic tolerance may be overcome by a trial of opioid dose escalation. On the contrary, opioid-induced pain could be worsened following an increase in opioid doses.

Opioid regimens and opioid-induced hyperalgesia

Several factors regarding an opioid regimen may influence the development of opioid-induced hyperalgesia. First of all, it remains to be investigated as to what opioid dose ranges lead to opioid-induced pain sensitivity. Opioid doses given through neuraxial or systemic routes in animal studies are comparable to moderate opioid doses in clinical settings. Second, there may be differences between different categories of opioid medications (eg, morphine versus methadone) in terms of their ability to induce hyperalgesia. Some evidence suggests that the development of opioid-induced hyperalgesia may differ between individual opioid medications [34]. Furthermore, is there cross pain sensitivity to other opioids following the treatment with one opioid? Last, the temporal correlation between opioid therapy and the development of opioid-induced hyperalgesia remains unknown, although opioid-induced hyperalgesia has been demonstrated in patients receiving a short intraoperative course of opioids. With a given dose of opioid treatment, how long would it take to develop opioid-induced hyperalgesia in a clinical setting? Conceivably opioid-induced pain sensitivity would be more likely to develop in patients receiving high opioid doses with a sustained treatment course.

Opioids and preemptive analgesia

While the clinical relevance and effectiveness of preemptive analgesia remains an issue in debate, several reasons may argue against the use of opioids as the main agent for preemptive analgesia. A large dose of intraoperative opioids may activate a pronociceptive system leading to the development of hyperalgesia postoperatively. This may confound the postoperative pain assessment and counteract the opioid analgesic effects. Also, the idea of preemptive analgesia calls for preemptive inhibition of neural plastic changes largely mediated through the activation of the central glutamatergic system. Opioids are thought to inhibit the nociceptive input that could activate the central glutamatergic system. However, neural mechanisms of opioid tolerance and opioid-induced hyperalgesia may interact with those of pathological pain and pathological pain could be exacerbated with opioid administration [41].

Approach to a patient on opioid regimen with increased pain

In evaluating a patient receiving opioid treatment who has increased pain, it is important to systematically review the various aspects of the "differential diagnosis" stated above. Once increased nociceptive activities (eg, disease progression) or psychological processes have been ruled out as the primary contributors to the patient's worsened pain, one is left with the task of differentiating between pharmacologic tolerance and opioid-induced hyperalgesia. It will not be unreasonable to give a trial of opioid dose escalation at this point. If the patient's pain improves, the cause of the pain is more likely to be tolerance. However, if the patient's pain worsens or does not consistently respond to the dose escalation, it could be a result of opioid-induced hyperalgesia and the dose should be decreased or even weaned off. The patient may also exhibit other features of opioid-induced hyperalgesia as described previously, which can help confirm this diagnosis.

In addition, one can consider opioid rotation, as patients can get better relief of their pain using a different medication, often at lower equi-analgesic dosages. We also recommend using adjuvant pain medication treatments to minimize the amount of opioid the patient is taking, thereby reducing the risk of tolerance and hyperalgesia occurring. Last, one should also consider the history of the patient's pain and its responsiveness to opioids. A patient who was previously on a stable opioid regimen and now complains of worsening pain is much different than one whose pain never improved with opioids. In the latter case, the patient should be weaned off the opioid and a nonopioid regimen pursued, instead of having continued dose escalations.

Differentiation of related phenomena in the context of opioid therapy

Physical dependence occurs when there is a withdrawal syndrome after abrupt cessation or dose reduction of the opioid or after administration of an antagonist drug [1]. Physical dependence is a reflection of neurophysiologic adaptation, thought to occur at peripheral and central neurons as a result of changes induced in opioid receptors [42]. Some of the signs and symptoms of withdrawal are listed below.

Symptoms of withdrawal: restlessness, irritability, increased sensitivity to pain, craving for opioids, nausea, abdominal cramps, myalgias, dysphoria, anxiety, insomnia.

Signs of withdrawal: sweating, piloerection, tachycardia, vomiting, diarrhea, hypertension, papillary dilation, yawning, fever, rhinorrhea.

It is not known clinically as to how long or what dose can increase a patient's likelihood of developing physical dependence. It should be assumed that the patient is predisposed after repeated doses over several days. Patients on opioids for a short period (several weeks) followed with the cessation of administration may often have very mild withdrawal symptoms that they do not recognize. Patients on long-acting opioids, such as methadone, can also have mild withdrawal symptoms even with abrupt cessation because of slow elimination. Severe withdrawal symptoms can, however, be precipitated with administration of naloxone, an opioid antagonist. Indeed, symptoms can occur even in individuals after one to two doses of an opioid, with no history of opioid dependence [43].

The withdrawal symptoms, although extremely unpleasant, are not considered to be life threatening. However, it is the fear of withdrawal that is a positive reinforcer both for continued self-administration of morphine in animals [44] and for continued drug-seeking behavior in patients who try to avoid these symptoms. It is important to note that physical dependence and this type of drug-seeking behavior do not necessarily indicate addiction.

Addiction is defined as a behavioral pattern of drug use, characterized by overwhelming involvement with the use of a drug (compulsive use), the securing of its supply, and the high tendency to relapse after withdrawal [42]. It is a group of maladaptive behaviors, including loss of control, preoccupation with drug use, and results in adverse consequences of use. Addiction is distinct from physical dependence and it should be noted that addiction is a psychological and behavioral process.

Pseudoaddiction describes an iatrogenic syndrome of behavioral changes that is similar to addiction, but develops as a result of inadequate pain management [45]. Severe and uncontrolled pain can result in increasing demands and drug-seeking behavior from the patient. This behavior may result in increasing suspicions on the part of the clinician that the patient is "addicted" and unwillingness to provide more opioids. The patient then becomes increasingly angry and distrustful of the clinician because of the inadequate treatment of the pain as well as the suspicions of addiction. It is important for the clinician to be aware of this syndrome and continually reevaluate the patient's clinical status with alterations in the therapeutic management.

The evidence of the development of addiction in patients with chronic administration of opioids has been mixed. Several studies have not shown abnormal drug-seeking behavior in patients with post-herpetic neuralgia, phantom limb pain, and chronic spinal pain [3]. But another study by Maruta and colleagues [46] showed that 65% of 144 consecutive patients referred for chronic nonmalignant pain management were abusing or "dependent on" weak and strong opioid drugs and had a strong family history of alcohol abuse. Because of the wide range of responses to opioid therapy in chronic pain patients, Portenoy [47] has suggested redefining addiction in these patients as

(1) an intense desire for the drug and overwhelming concern about its continued availability (psychological dependence);
(2) evidence of compulsive drug use (characterized, for example, by unsanctioned dose escalation, continued dosing despite significant side effects, use of drug to treat symptoms not targeted by therapy, or unapproved use during period of no symptoms); or
(3) evidence of one or more of a group of associated behaviors, including manipulation of the treating physician or medical system for the purposes of obtaining additional drug (altering prescriptions, for example), acquisition of drugs from other medical sources or from a nonmedical source, drug hoarding or sales, or unapproved use of other drugs (particularly alcohol or other sedatives/hypnotics) during opioid therapy.

Abuse describes the use of a medication by the patient in a way that may cause harm to him- or herself or to others, or the use of the medication for an indication other than that intended by the prescribing clinician. An abuser may or may not be physically dependent or addicted to the opioid [42].

Summary

In summary, the phenomena of opioid tolerance and opioid-induced hyperalgesia have been well documented and contribute to the decreased analgesic efficacy of opioids. In the clinical setting, patient reports of increased pain require a systematic approach in consideration of the possible etiologies. In addition, there should be awareness that increasing the opioid dose may not always be the answer. Under certain circumstances, less opioid may be more effective in pain reduction. This approach may be combined with opioid rotation or addition of nonopioid adjuvant medications. In addition, opioid tolerance and opioid-induced hyperalgesia need to be differentiated from physical dependence, addiction, pseudoaddiction, and abuse.

References

[1] Jaffe JH. Drug addiction and drug abuse. In: Gilman AG, Goodman LS, Rall TW, et al, editors. The pharmacological basis of therapeutics. 7th edition. New York: Macmillan; 1985. p. 532–81.
[2] O'Brien CP. Drug addiction and drug abuse. In: Hardman JG, Limbird LE, editors. Goodman and Gilman's the pharmacological basis of therapeutics. 9th edition. New York: McGraw-Hill; 1995. p. 557–77.
[3] Collett B-J. Opioid tolerance: the clinical perspective. Br J Anaesth 1998;81:58–68.
[4] Arner S, Rawal N, Gustafsson LL. Clinical experience of long-term treatment with epidural and intrathecal opioids—a nationwide survery. Acta Anaesthesiol Scand 1988;32(3):253–9.

[5] Cochin J, Kornetsky C. Development and loss of tolerance to morphine in the rat after single and multiple injections. J Pharmacol Exp Ther 1964;145:1–20.

[6] Yaksh TL. Tolerance: factors involved in changes in the dose-effect relationship with chronic drug exposure. In: Basbaum AI, Besson J-M, editors. Towards a new pharmacotherapy of pain. Chichester: John Wiley & Sons; 1991. p. 157–79.

[7] Sosnowski M, Yaksh TL. Differential cross-tolerance between intrathecal morphine and sufentanil in the rat. Anesthesiology 1990;73:1141–7.

[8] Stevens CW, Yaksh TL. Studies of morphine and D-ala-D-leu-enkephalin (DADLE) cross-tolerance after continuous intrathecal infusion in the rat. Anesthesiology 1992;76:596–603.

[9] Fernandes M, Kluwe S, Coper H. The development of tolerance to morphine in the rat. Psychopharmacology (Berl) 1977a;54(2):197–201.

[10] Fernandes M, Kluwe S, Coper H. Quantitative assessment of tolerance to and dependence on morphine in mice. Naunyn Schmiedebergs Arch Pharmacol 1997b;297(1):53–60.

[11] Yaksh TL, Kohl RL, Rudy TA. Induction of tolerance and withdrawal in rats receiving morphine in the spinal subarachnoid space. Eur J Pharmacol 1977;42(3):275–84.

[12] Roerig SC, Fujimoto JM. Morphine antinociception in different strains of mice: relationship of supraspinal-spinal multiplicative interaction to tolerance. J Pharmacol Exp Ther 1988;247(2):603–8.

[13] Woolf CJ. Intrathecal high dose morphine produces hyperalgesia in the rat. Brain Res 1981;209(2):491–5.

[14] Yaksh TL, Harty GJ, Onofrio BM. High dose of spinal morphine produces a nonopiate receptor-mediated hyperesthesia: clinical and theoretic implications. Anesthesiology 1986;64(5):590–7.

[15] Mao J. Opioid-induced abnormal pain sensitivity: Is it clinically relevant? Curr Pain Headache Rep 2006;10(1):67–70.

[16] Mao J, Price DD, Mayer DJ. Thermal hyperalgesia in association with the development of morphine tolerance in rats: roles of excitatory amino acid receptors and protein kinase C. J Neurosci 1994;14:2301–12.

[17] Mao J, Sung B, Ji RR, et al. Chronic morphine induces downregulation of spinal glutamate transporters: implication sin morphine tolerance and abnormal pain sensitivity. J Neurosci 2002;22:8312–23.

[18] Mao J, Sung B, Ji RR, et al. Neuronal apoptosis associated with morphine tolerance: evidence for an opioid-induced neurotoxic mechanism. J Neurosci 2002;22:7650–61.

[19] Celerier E, Rivat C, Jun Y, et al. Long lasting hyperalgesia induced by fentanyl in rats: preventive effect of ketamine. Anesthesiology 2000;92:465–72.

[20] Laulin JP, Maurette P, Corcuff JB, et al. The role of ketamine in preventing fentanyl-induced hyperalgesia and subsequent acute morphine tolerance. Anesth Analg 2002;94:1263–9.

[21] Celerier E, Laulin JP, Corcuff JB, et al. Progressive enhancement of delayed hyperalgesia induced by repeated heroin administration: a sensitization process. J Neurosci 2001;21:4074–80.

[22] Vanderah TW, Ossipov MH, Lai J, et al. Mechanisms of opioid induced pain and antinociceptive tolerance: descending facilitation and spinal dynorphin. Pain 2001;92:5–9.

[23] Vinik HR, Igor K. Rapid development of tolerance to analgesia during remifentanil infusion in humans. Anesth Analg 1998;86:307–11.

[24] Crawford MW, Hickey C, Zaarour C, et al. Development of acute opioid tolerance during infusion of remifentanil for pediatric scoliosis surgery. Anesth Analg 2006;102(6):1662–7.

[25] Guignard B, Bossard AE, Coste C, et al. Acute opioid tolerance: intraoperative remifentanil increases postoperative pain and morphine requiremnt. Anesthesiology 2000;93(2):409–17.

[26] Gourlay GK, Plummer JL, Cheery DA, et al. Comparison of intermittent bolus with continuous infusion of epidural morphine in the treatment of severe cancer pain. Pain 1991;47:135–40.

[27] Penn RD, Paice JA. Chronic intrathecal morphine for intractable pain. J Neurosurg 1987;67:182–6.

[28] Mahowald ML, Singh JA, Majeski P. Opioid use by patients in an orthopedics spine clinic. Arthritis Rheum 2005;52(1):312–21.

[29] Chu LF, Clark DJ, Angst MS. Opioid tolerance and hyperalgesia in chronic pain patients after one month of oral morphine therapy: a preliminary prospective study. J Pain 2006; 7(1):43–8.

[30] Bruera E, MacMillan K, Hanson J, et al. The cognitive effects of the administration of narcotic analgesics in patients with cancer pain. Pain 1989;39:13–6.

[31] Ho A, Dole VP. Pain perception in drug-free and in methadone-maintained human ex-addicts. Proc Soc Exp Biol Med 1979;162:392–5.

[32] Compton P, Charuvastra VC, Kintaudi K, et al. Pain responses in methadone-maintained opioid abusers. J Pain Symptom Manage 2000;20:237–45.

[33] Doverty M, White JM, Somogyi AA, et al. Hyperalgesic responses in methadone maintenance patients. Pain 2001;90:91–6.

[34] Compton P, Charuvastra VC, Ling W. Pain intolerance in opioid-maintained former opiate addicts: effect of long-acting maintenance agent. Drug Alcohol Depend 2001;63:139–46.

[35] Wilson GR, Reisfield GM. Morphine hyperalgesia: a case report. Am J Hosp Palliat Care 2003;20(6):459–61.

[36] Mercadante S, Ferrera P, Villari P, et al. Hyperalgesia: an emerging iatrogenic syndrome. J Pain Symptom Manage 2003;26(2):769–75.

[37] Heger S, Maier C, Otter K, et al. Morphine induced allodynia in a child with brain tumour. BMJ 1999;319(7210):627–9.

[38] Sjogren P, Jensen NH, Jensen TS. Disappearance of morphine-induced hyperalgesia after discontinuing or substituting morphine with opioid agonists. Pain 1994;59:313–6.

[39] Ossipov MH, Lai J, Vanderah TW, et al. Induction of pain facilitation by sustained opioid exposure: relationship to opioid antinociceptive tolerance. Life Sci 2003;73:783–800.

[40] Portenoy RK. Tolerance to opioid analgesics: clinical aspects. Cancer Surv 1994;21:49–65.

[41] Mao J, Price DD, Mayer DJ. Mechanisms of hyperalgesia and opioid tolerance: a current view of their possible interactions. Pain 1995;62:259–74.

[42] Savage SR. Opioid use in the management of chronic pain. Med Clin North Am 1999;83(3): 761–86.

[43] Jaffe JH. Misinformation: euphoria and addiction. In: Hill CS Jr, Fields WS, editors. Advances in pain research and therapy. Vol 11. New York: Raven Press; 1989. p. 163–73.

[44] Lyness WH, Smith RL, Heavner JE, et al. Morphine self-administration in the rat during adjuvant arthritis. Life Sci 1989;45:2217–24.

[45] Weissman DE, Haddox JD. Opioid pseudoaddiction: an iatrogenic syndrome. Pain 1989;36: 363–6.

[46] Maruta T, Swanson DW, Finlayson RE. Drug abuse and dependency in patients with chronic pain. Mayo Clin Proc 1979;54:241–4.

[47] Portenoy RK. Chronic opioid therapy in nonmalignant pain. J Pain Symptom Manage 1990; 5:S46–62.

THE MEDICAL
CLINICS
OF NORTH AMERICA

Med Clin N Am 91 (2007) 213–228

Documentation and Potential Tools in Long-Term Opioid Therapy for Pain

Howard S. Smith, MD, FACP[a],*,
Kenneth L. Kirsh, PhD[b]

[a]Albany Medical College, Department of Anesthesiology, 47 New Scotland Avenue,
MC-131 Albany, New York 12208, USA
[b]Pharmacy Practice and Science, University of Kentucky, 725 Rose Street, 401C,
Lexington, KY 40536-0082, USA

Tremendous progress has been made in the study and treatment of pain in the past 2 decades [1,2]. Efforts have been undertaken to make pain assessment and treatment a priority of medical care and to use all of the weapons in our arsenal to bring relief to the millions of people with chronic pain [3,4]. However, this progress has been somewhat tempered by the souring of the regulatory climate and the growth of prescription drug abuse. Because of this, there has been a trend for clinicians to shy away from using high opioid doses or even using this modality at all in the treatment of chronic pain [5–7].

Despite these setbacks, the use of long-term opioid therapy (LTOT) to treat chronic noncancer pain is growing, based in part on evidence from clinical trials and a growing consensus among pain specialists [8–12]. The appropriate use of these drugs requires skills in opioid prescribing, knowledge of addiction medicine principles, and a commitment to perform and document a comprehensive assessment repeatedly over time. Inadequate assessment can lead to undertreatment, compromise the effectiveness of therapy when implemented, and prevent an appropriate response when problematic drug-related behaviors occur [13–15].

Fortunately, there is a growing interest in the development of tools that can be useful for screening patients up front to determine relative risk for patients having problems with prescription drug abuse or misuse. Regarding brief screening instruments, a number have arisen, including the Screening Tool for Addiction Risk (STAR) [16], Drug Abuse Screening Test (DAST) [17], Screener and Opioid Assessment for Patients with Pain (SOAPP) [18], and the Opioid Risk Tool (ORT) [19] among others. The

* Corresponding author.
E-mail address: SmithH@mail.amc.edu (H.S. Smith).

choice in tools for more thorough ongoing assessment, however, has been somewhat more limited up until now and will be the focus of our discussion.

Regulatory agencies, state medical boards, and various peer-review groups among others not only expect appropriate medical care but also require proper documentation. In cases of LTOT for chronic pain, aside from the usual "SOAP" (ie, subjective/objective/assessment/plan)-style medical progress notes, various other issues may deserve documentation. Although there are no explicit requirements spelled out as to what and how to document issues related to LTOT, it is felt by some that the use of specific tools/ instruments in the chart on some or all visits may boost adherence to documentation expectations as well as consistency of such documentation. Assessment tools may also be helpful in the analysis of persistent pain [20].

It must be cautioned that physicians who adequately assess patients before and during opioid therapy may still encounter problems as a result of poor documentation. In a chart review of 300 patients with chronic pain, 61% had no documentation of a treatment plan [21]. Similarly, a review of the initial consultation notes of 513 patients with acute musculoskeletal pain revealed that only 43% of historical findings and 28% of physical examination findings were documented [22]. In a review of 520 randomly selected visits at an outpatient oncology practice, quantitative assessment of pain scores occurred in less than 1% of cases and qualitative assessment of pain occurred in only 60% of cases [23]. Finally, a review of medical records of 111 randomly selected patients who underwent urine toxicology screens in a cancer center found that documentation was infrequent: 37.8% of physicians failed to list a reason for the test, and 89% of the charts did not include the results of the test [24].

Areas of interest for documentation

Clearly, strategies are needed to translate these recommendations for patient assessment during long-term opioid therapy to frontline practice. This effort would certainly benefit from the availability of a consistent method of documentation. As one potential framework, it is important to consider four main domains in assessing pain outcomes and to better protect your practice for those patients you maintain on an opioid regimen: (1) pain relief, (2) functional outcomes, (3) side effects, and (4) drug-related behaviors. These domains have been labeled the "Four A's" (Analgesia, Activities of daily living, Adverse effects, and Aberrant drug-related behaviors) for teaching purposes [25]. There are, of course, many different ways to think about these domains, and multiple attempts to capture them will be discussed in this article.

The Pain Assessment and Documentation Tool

The Pain Assessment and Documentation Tool (PADT) is a simple charting device based on the 4 A's concept that is designed to focus on key outcomes and provide a consistent way to document progress in pain management therapy over time. Twenty-seven clinicians completed the preliminary version of the PADT for 388 opioid-treated patients [26,27]. Nineteen clinicians (17 physicians, 1 nurse, and 1 psychologist) participated in a debriefing phase. Twelve of the 19 clinicians had participated in the field trial before the debriefing. The debriefing interview for these clinicians used the same standard questions to evaluate both the original and revised PADT.

The result of this work is a brief, two-sided chart note that can be readily included in the patient's medical record. It was designed to be intuitive, pragmatic, and adaptable to clinical situations. In the field trial, it took clinicians between 10 and 20 minutes to complete the tool. The revised PADT is substantially shorter and should require a few minutes to complete. By addressing the need for documentation, the PADT can assist clinicians in meeting their obligations for ongoing assessment and documentation. Although the PADT is not intended to replace a progress note, it is well suited to complement existing documentation with a focused evaluation of outcomes that are clinically relevant and address the need for evidence of appropriate monitoring.

The decision to assess the four domains subsumed under the shorthand designation, the "Four A's," was based on clinical experience, the positive comments received by the investigators during educational programs on opioid pharmacotherapy for noncancer pain, and an evolving national movement that recognizes the need to approach opioid therapy with a "balanced" response. This response recognizes both the legitimate need to provide optimal therapy to appropriate patients and the need to acknowledge the potential for abuse, diversion, and addiction [25]. The value of assessing pain relief, side effects, and aspects of functioning has been emphasized repeatedly in the literature [21,28–31]. Documentation of drug-related behaviors is a relatively new concept that is being explored for the first time in the PADT.

Assessing opioid therapy adverse effects

Documentation of adverse effects in a majority of charts from many pain clinics tend to be addressed (or in many cases not addressed) in their charts by a brief note of the presence or absence of one or more adverse effects (eg, nausea, constipation, itching), noted by busy clinicians. Similar to the goal of the PADT, having a standardized form that is used at every visit and filled out by the patients before being seen by health care providers may provide certain advantages.

Patients with persistent pain on oral opioid therapy have asked to "come off" the opioids because of adverse effects, even if they perceived that opioids were providing reasonable analgesic effects [32]. The distress that may be caused by opioid adverse effects may also be seen with acute postoperative pain patients, who may occasionally ask to stop their opioids despite that they are perceived as effective analgesics, because of the significant distress and suffering that they perceive they are experiencing from an opioid adverse effect.

It therefore appears crucial to assess opioid adverse effects. Ideally, this should be done in a manner as to be able to follow trends as well as compare the patients' perceived intensity of the adverse effects versus the intensity of pain or other symptoms or adverse effects.

One available tool for the quantification of adverse effects is the Numerical Opioid Side Effect (NOSE) assessment tool (see Fig. 1) [33]. The NOSE instrument is self-administered, can be completed by the patient in minutes, and can be entered into electronic databases or inserted into a hard-copy chart on each patient visit. The NOSE assessment tool is easy to administer as well as easy to interpret and may provide clinicians with important clinical information that could potentially impact various therapeutic decisions. Although most clinicians probably routinely assess adverse effects of treatments, it is sometimes difficult to find legible, clear, and concise documentation of such information in outpatient records. Furthermore, the documentation that does exist may not always attempt to "quantify" the intensity of treatment-related adverse effects or lend itself to looking at trends.

	Not Present									As Bad As You Can Imagine	
	0	1	2	3	4	5	6	7	8	9	10
1. Nausea, vomiting, and/or lack of appetite	O	O	O	O	O	O	O	O	O	O	O
2. Fatigue, sleepiness, trouble concentrating, hallucinations, and/or drowsiness/somnolence	O	O	O	O	O	O	O	O	O	O	O
3. Constipation	O	O	O	O	O	O	O	O	O	O	O
4. Itching	O	O	O	O	O	O	O	O	O	O	O
5. Decreased sexual desire/function and/or diminished libido	O	O	O	O	O	O	O	O	O	O	O
6. Dry Mouth	O	O	O	O	O	O	O	O	O	O	O
7. Abdominal pain or discomfort/cramping or bloating	O	O	O	O	O	O	O	O	O	O	O
8. Sweating	O	O	O	O	O	O	O	O	O	O	O
9. Headache and/or dizziness	O	O	O	O	O	O	O	O	O	O	O
10. Urinary retention	O	O	O	O	O	O	O	O	O	O	O

Fig. 1. Numerical Opioid Side Effect (NOSE) assessment tool.

Assessing LTOT efficacy

The Initiative on Methods, Measurements, and Pain Assessment in Clinical Trials (IMMPACT) recommended that six core outcome domains ([1] pain, [2] physical functions, [3] emotion, [4] participant rating of improvement and satisfaction with treatment, [5] symptoms and adverse events, and [6] participant disposition) should be considered when designing chronic pain clinical trials [34]. The authors believe that the use of a unidimensional tool such as the numerical rating scale-11 (NRS-11) provides a suboptimal assessment of chronic pain as well as LTOT efficacy. Clinicians should attempt to assess multiple domains (preferably with multidimensional tools) in efforts to achieve a global picture of the patient's baseline status as well as the patient's response to LTOT in various domains.

It has been proposed that the use of a collection of various tools may provide adjunct information and help clinicians to create a more complete picture regarding longitudinal trends of overall progress/functioning for their patients with chronic pain on LTOT [35]. Assessing individual outcomes during outpatient multidisciplinary chronic pain treatment is often an extremely challenging task. There are many tools and instruments currently available, but the Treatment Outcomes in Pain Survey tool (TOPS) has been specifically designed to assess and follow outcomes in the chronic pain population and has been described as an augmented SF-36 [36,37]. The Medical Outcomes Study (MOS) Short Form 36-item questionnaire (SF-36) compares the health status of large populations without a preponderance of one single medical condition [38]. The SF-36 assesses eight domains, but it has not been found to be especially useful for following the changes in function and pain in chronic pain populations.

The eight domains of the SF-36 are bodily pain (BP), general health (GH), mental health (MH), physical functioning (PF), role emotional (RE), social functioning (SF), role physical (RP), and vitality (VT). The TOPS scale initially had nine domains, but one (satisfaction with outcomes) was modified in subsequent versions. The nine domains of TOPS are Pain Symptom, Family/Social Disability, Functional Limitations, Total Pain Experience, Objective Work Disability, Life Control, Solicitous Responses, Passive Coping, and Satisfaction with Outcomes. This enhanced SF-36 (TOPS scale) was constructed by obtaining patient data from the SF-36 with 12 additional role-functioning questions. These additional questions were taken in part from the 61-item Multidimensional Pain Inventory (MPI) [39] and the 10-item Oswestry Disability Questionnaire [40], with four additional pain-related questions that are similar to those found in the MOS pain-related questions [41], the Brief Pain Inventory [28], and a six-item coping scale from the MOS [41].

The question adapted from the Oswestry Disability Questionnaire (designed for back pain patients) includes questions that relate to impairment (pain), physical functioning (how long the patient can sit or stand), and disability (ability to travel or have sexual relations) [40]. The patient-generated index is an instrument that attempts to individualize a patient's perception of his or her quality of life [42].

Although the TOPS instrument is an extremely useful tool, it is time-consuming, is based entirely on the patient's subjective responses, and requires that the clinician has access, whether by a special computer program or by sending forms away, for scoring. As a result, it may not be an ideal instrument to use in every pain clinic and may not provide the clinician with an answer immediately of how the patient is doing relative to previous visits (although it may have that potential with adequate time, scanning equipment, and computer software).

Translational analgesia

A concept that may possess potential utility for clinicians is translational analgesia. Translational analgesia refers to improvements in physical, social, or emotional function that are realized by the patient as a result of improved analgesia, or essentially what did the pain relief experienced by the patient "translate" into in terms of perceived improved quality of life [43]. In most cases, a sustained and significant improvement in pain perception that is deemed worthwhile to the patient should "translate" into improvement in quality of life or improved social, emotional, or physical function. Improvements in social, emotional, or physical domains are often spontaneously reported by patients, but in most cases should be able to be ascertained or elicited via "focused" interview techniques with the patient, significant others, and family; "focused" physical exam; or a combination of any of these. Improvements may be subtle and could include a range of daily function activities or other signs (eg, going out more with friends, doing laundry, showing improved mood/relations with family members). It is important to note that this issue is certainly not exclusive to opioid therapy and is thought to apply to other treatments.

The authors do not deem it inappropriate or inhumane to taper relatively "high-dose" opioid therapy in a patient with chronic pain who notes that his or her NRS-11 "pain score" has dropped from 9/10 to 8/10 after escalating to over a gram of long-acting morphine preparation per day but in whom the patient as well as the patient's family or significant other cannot describe (and the clinician cannot elicit) any significant "translational analgesia." A patient with chronic pain who demonstrates a failure to "get off the couch," despite equivocal or minimally improved analgesia, should not be considered as a therapeutic success. But, should this viewpoint be seen as cruel or as a punishment for these patients? Rome and colleagues [44] demonstrated that at least a subpopulation of patients seems to do better after tapering off opioids. Furthermore, more evidence regarding the hyperalgesic actions of opioids in certain circumstances is mounting [45,46].

The periodic assessment of the patient with chronic pain should be performed in multiple domains (eg, social domain, analgesia domain, functional domain, emotional domain). The authors believe the relatively common practice of evaluating patients with chronic pain by obtaining an NRS-11 pain score at each assessment and basing opioid analgesic treatment solely on this score to be suboptimal. Although tools exist that assess multiple domains used in research, there is no simple, convenient, and universally acceptable instrument that is used in busy clinical pain practices.

To address this issue, a recent tool has been developed. The SAFE score (see section titled "The SAFE score") is a multidomain assessment tool that may have potential utility for rapid dynamic assessment in the busy clinic setting [47,48]. The SAFE score is a clinician-generated tool and may best be used in conjunction with the translational analgesic score (TAS) (a patient-generated tool) as an adjunct. These are discussed, in turn, in the following two sections.

The translational analgesic score

The translational analgesic score (TAS) is a patient-generated tool that attempts to quantify the degree of "translational analgesia" (see Fig. 2) [48]. It is simple, rapid, user-friendly, and suitable for use in busy pain clinics. The patient can be handed the TAS sheet with questions to fill out at each visit while in the waiting room and the responses are averaged for an overall score that is recorded in the chart. The authors encourage clinicians to have all patients write down specific examples of things that they can now do or do frequently that they couldn't do or did rarely when their pain was less controlled. Alternatively, the patients' responses can be entered into a computerized record (with graphs of trends) if the pain clinic's medical records are electronic.

In the sample provided, the patient answered all 10 questions with responses, hence, the average is the sum of all responses (26) divided by 10. Therefore, the TAS is 2.6. A patient, who at each visit consistently has a TAS of 10.0, clearly represents a therapeutic success on their current treatment. Conversely, a patient who at each visit consistently has a TAS of 0.0 would represent a suboptimal therapeutic result (by TAS criteria). Clinicians are encouraged to document at least one or two specific examples of translational analgesia (eg, perhaps various activities that the patient can now perform as a result of pain relief or can now perform frequently as a result of pain relief that the patient could not do or only do infrequently before therapy) on the bottom or reverse side of the TAS score sheet. Treatment decisions regarding escalation or tapering of opioids, changing agents, adding agents, obtaining consultations, instituting physical medicine or behavioral medicine techniques, remain the medical judgment of practitioners and should be based on a careful reevaluation of the patient and not based on a number.

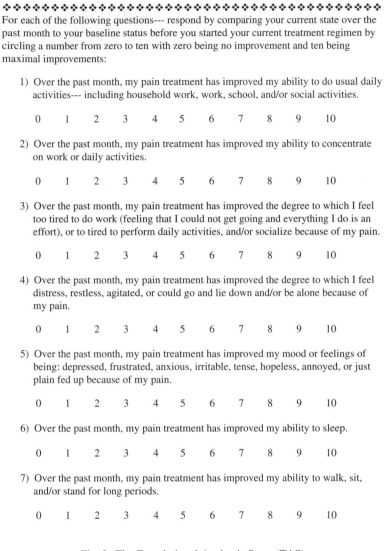

❖ ❖
For each of the following questions--- respond by comparing your current state over the
past month to your baseline status before you started your current treatment regimen by
circling a number from zero to ten with zero being no improvement and ten being
maximal improvements:

1) Over the past month, my pain treatment has improved my ability to do usual daily
   activities--- including household work, work, school, and/or social activities.

   0   1   2   3   4   5   6   7   8   9   10

2) Over the past month, my pain treatment has improved my ability to concentrate
   on work or daily activities.

   0   1   2   3   4   5   6   7   8   9   10

3) Over the past month, my pain treatment has improved the degree to which I feel
   too tired to do work (feeling that I could not get going and everything I do is an
   effort), or to tired to perform daily activities, and/or socialize because of my pain.

   0   1   2   3   4   5   6   7   8   9   10

4) Over the past month, my pain treatment has improved the degree to which I feel
   distress, restless, agitated, or could go and lie down and/or be alone because of
   my pain.

   0   1   2   3   4   5   6   7   8   9   10

5) Over the past month, my pain treatment has improved my mood or feelings of
   being: depressed, frustrated, anxious, irritable, tense, hopeless, annoyed, or just
   plain fed up because of my pain.

   0   1   2   3   4   5   6   7   8   9   10

6) Over the past month, my pain treatment has improved my ability to sleep.

   0   1   2   3   4   5   6   7   8   9   10

7) Over the past month, my pain treatment has improved my ability to walk, sit,
   and/or stand for long periods.

   0   1   2   3   4   5   6   7   8   9   10

Fig. 2. The Translational Analgesic Score (TAS).

8) Over the past month, my pain treatment has improved my ability to go up stairs, and/or move or lift objects.

    0   1   2   3   4   5   6   7   8   9   10

9) Over the past month, my pain treatment has improved the extent to which my pain interferes with optimal interpersonal relationships and/or intimacy.

    0   1   2   3   4   5   6   7   8   9   10

10) Over the past month, to what degree have you, your significant other, your family, your co-workers, and/or your friends noticed any improvements in your socializing, recreational activities, physical functioning, concentration, mood, interpersonal relationships, activities of daily living, and/or overall quality of life?

    0   1   2   3   4   5   6   7   8   9   10

--- Please write below--- specific examples of things you can now do or currently do frequently that you couldn't do or only did rarely when your pain was not controlled as well as it is now.

TAS = _____

❖ ❖

The TAS is expressed as a number between 0 to 10 with a decimal being the average of the responses to the ten questions (or less--- if the patient is paraplegic then they would not answer the questions regarding going up stairs, etc.).

As an example, a patient's response to the TAS tool is shown below:
1) Over the past month, my pain treatment has improved my ability to do usual daily activities--- including household work, work, school, and/or social activities.

    0   1   2   3   •   5   6   7   8   9   10

2) Over the past month, my pain treatment has improved my ability to concentrate on work or daily activities.

    0   1   2   •   4   5   6   7   8   9   10

3) Over the past month, my pain treatment has improved the degree to which I feel too tired to do work (feeling that I could not get going and everything I do is an effort), or to tired to perform daily activities, and/or socialize because of my pain.

    0   1   2   •   4   5   6   7   8   9   10

Fig. 2 (*continued*)

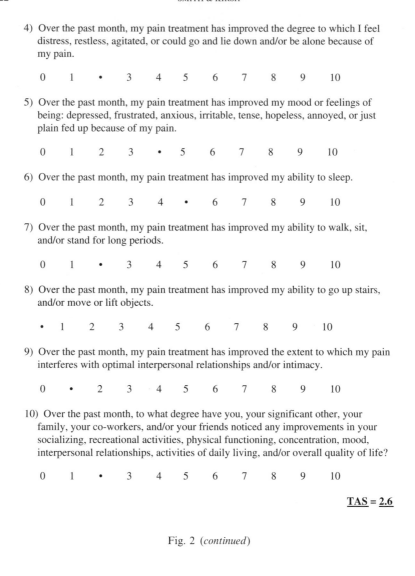

4) Over the past month, my pain treatment has improved the degree to which I feel distress, restless, agitated, or could go and lie down and/or be alone because of my pain.

    0   1   •   3   4   5   6   7   8   9   10

5) Over the past month, my pain treatment has improved my mood or feelings of being: depressed, frustrated, anxious, irritable, tense, hopeless, annoyed, or just plain fed up because of my pain.

    0   1   2   3   •   5   6   7   8   9   10

6) Over the past month, my pain treatment has improved my ability to sleep.

    0   1   2   3   4   •   6   7   8   9   10

7) Over the past month, my pain treatment has improved my ability to walk, sit, and/or stand for long periods.

    0   1   •   3   4   5   6   7   8   9   10

8) Over the past month, my pain treatment has improved my ability to go up stairs, and/or move or lift objects.

    •   1   2   3   4   5   6   7   8   9   10

9) Over the past month, my pain treatment has improved the extent to which my pain interferes with optimal interpersonal relationships and/or intimacy.

    0   •   2   3   4   5   6   7   8   9   10

10) Over the past month, to what degree have you, your significant other, your family, your co-workers, and/or your friends noticed any improvements in your socializing, recreational activities, physical functioning, concentration, mood, interpersonal relationships, activities of daily living, and/or overall quality of life?

    0   1   •   3   4   5   6   7   8   9   10

TAS = 2.6

Fig. 2 (*continued*)

The concept of translational analgesia is not meant to imply that opioids should be tapered, weaned, or discontinued. If a patient has a TAS that is very low and essentially unchanged over time (especially in conjunction with a SAFE score in the "red zone"), then this should prompt the clinician to reevaluate the patient and consider a change in therapy. This could mean pursuing various therapeutic options including perhaps increasing the dose of opioids. However, if a patient has a high TAS and a SAFE score in the green zone, the patient should probably continue LTOT.

The SAFE score

Another tool that has been advocated to help with this purpose is called the SAFE score [47,48]. Although it has not yet been rigorously validated, it is simple and practical and may possess clinical utility. It is a score generated by the health care provider that is meant to reflect a multidimensional assessment of outcome to opioid therapy. It is not meant to replace more elaborate patient-based assessment tools but could possibly serve as an adjunct and possibly in the future shed some light on the difference between patients' perception of how they are doing on opioid treatment versus the physician-based view of outcome.

At each visit, the clinician rates the patient's functioning and pain relief in four domains. The domains assessed include social functioning (S), analgesia or pain relief (A), physical functioning (F), and emotional functioning (E). Together, the ratings in each of the four domains are combined to yield a "SAFE" score. The "SAFE" score can range from 4 to 20.

The SAFE tool is both practical in its ease and clinically useful (Fig. 3). The goals of the SAFE tool are multifold. Specifically, they include the need to demonstrate that the clinician has routinely evaluated the efficacy of the treatment from multiple perspectives; guide the clinician toward a broader view of treatment options beyond adjusting the medication regimen; and

	Rating	Criterion				
Social Marital, family, friends, leisure, recreational		1 supportive harmonious socializing engaged	2	3	4	5 conflictual discord isolated bored
Analgesia Intensity, frequency, duration		1 comfortable effective controlled	2	3	4	5 intolerable ineffective uncontrolled
Function Work, ADL's, home management, school, training, physical activity		1 independent active productive energetic	2	3	4	5 dependent unmotivated passive deconditioned
Emotional Cognitive, stress, attitude, mood, behavior, neuro-vegetative signs		1 clear relaxed optimistic upbeat composed	2	3	4	5 confused tense pessimistic depressed distressed
Total Score						

The patient's status in each of the four domains is rated as follows:

1 = Excellent
2 = Good
3 = Fair
4 = Borderline
5 = Poor

Fig. 3. Sample SAFE form.

document the clinician's rationale for continuation, modification, or cessation of opioid therapy.

Interpretation of scores

Scores can be broken down into three distinct categories. First, the *green zone* represents a SAFE score of 4 to 12 or decrease of 2 points in total score from baseline. With a score in the green zone, the patient is considered to be doing well and the plan would be to continue with the current medication regimen or consider reducing the total dose of the opioids. Second, the *yellow zone* represents a SAFE score of 13 to 16 or a rating of 5 in any category or an increase of 2 or more from baseline in the total score. With a score in the yellow zone, the patient should be monitored closely and reassessed frequently. Finally, the *red zone* represents a SAFE score greater than or equal to 17. With a score in the red zone, a change in the treatment would be warranted.

Once the color determination is made, a decision can be made regarding treatment options. Treatment options depend on the pattern of scores. If attempts are made to address problems in specific domains and the patient is still not showing an improvement in the SAFE score, then the patient may not be an appropriate candidate for long-term opioid therapy.

Fig. 4 illustrates green zone cases. In example A, there is good analgesic response to opioids, with a fair response in the other domains. No change in treatment would be necessary unless adverse reactions to the medications require an adjustment or discontinuation. In example B, there is borderline analgesic response, but good social and emotional responses and a fair physical functioning response. Some pain specialists may determine that the medication regimen should be optimized. For others, this pattern of ratings may reflect a reasonable improvement in quality of life for the patient. Therefore, continuing the present medication regimen would be a reasonable option.

Fig. 5 illustrates how the SAFE tool can be used to track changes in the status of the same patient on two consecutive visits. In the change in scores from example C to example D, although analgesia deteriorates from fair to borderline, there is significant improvement in the other domains. The clinician may feel this is satisfactory for this particular patient and continue with

Example A		Example B	
Social	3	Social	2
Analgesia	2	Analgesia	4
Function	3	Function	3
Emotional	3	Emotional	1
Green Zone "SAFE" score	11	*Green Zone* "SAFE" score	10

Fig. 4. Green zone cases using the SAFE scoring tool.

Example C

Social	5
Analgesia	3
Function	5
Emotional	5
Red Zone "SAFE" score	18

Example D

Social	3
Analgesia	4
Function	3
Emotional	3
Green Zone "SAFE" score	13

Fig. 5. Tracking an overall positive change in status using the SAFE scoring tool.

the current medication regimen. Once again, too narrow a focus on analgesic response may lead to unnecessary dose escalation. This case also illustrates the situation in which even though the total score at visit D is greater than 12 and would be a *yellow zone*, it is assigned as a *green zone* because there was a decrease of more than 2 in the total score. Alternately, the clinician may determine that a borderline analgesic response is not optimal. The choices for intervention may include rotating to another opioid agent, increasing the current opioid dose, adding adjuvant medications, referring for nonpharmacological treatment, or discontinuing high-dose opioids.

Fig. 6 illustrates again a single patient on two consecutive visits. Here, analgesia has remained good over time, but there has been a negative impact on the domains of function and emotion. Pain specialists who are focused on the pain scores of such a patient may be comfortable with continuing the established treatment plan. However, using SAFE, an expanded view of the patient's overall status will alert the clinician to monitor the patient's physical and emotional functioning in future visits. If the ratings in the psychological and physical domains persist, then the clinician may recommend that the patient pursue psychosocial treatment or physical rehabilitation in addition to maintaining the medication regimen.

Summary

Assessment and documentation are cornerstones for both protecting your practice and obtaining optimal patient outcomes while on opioid therapy. There are a growing number of assessment tools for clinicians to guide the evaluation of a group of important outcomes during opioid therapy

Example E

Social	3
Analgesia	2
Function	3
Emotional	3
Green Zone "SAFE" score	11

Example F

Social	3
Analgesia	2
Function	4
Emotional	4
Yellow Zone "SAFE" score	13

Fig. 6. Tracking an overall negative change in status using the SAFE scoring tool.

and provide a simple means of documenting patient care. They all have the capability to prove helpful in clinical management and offer mechanisms for documenting the types of practice standards that those in the regulatory and law enforcement communities seek to ensure.

References

[1] Berry PH, Dahl JL. The new JCAHO pain standards: implications for pain management nurses. Pain Manag Nurs 2000;1(1):3–12.
[2] SUPPORT Study Principal Investigators. A controlled trial to improve care for seriously ill hospitalized patients: a study to understand prognoses and preferences for outcomes and risks of treatment (SUPPORT). JAMA 1995;274:1591.
[3] Osterweis M, Kleinman A, Mechanic D, editors. Pain and disability: clinical, behavioral, and public policy perspectives. [Report of the Committee on Pain, Disability, and Chronic Illness Behavior, Institute of Medicine, National Academy of Sciences.] Washington, DC: National Academy Press; 1987.
[4] Verhaak PFM, Kerssens JJ, Dekker J, et al. Prevalence of chronic benign pain disorder among adults: a review of the literature. Pain 1998;77:231–9.
[5] Cicero TJ, Inciardi JA, Munoz A. Trends in abuse of Oxycontin and other opioid analgesics in the United States: 2002–2004. J Pain 2005;6(10):662–72.
[6] Lipman AG. Does the DEA truly seek balance in pain medicine? J Pain Palliat Care Pharmacother 2005;19(1):7–9.
[7] Passik SD, Kirsh KL. Fear and loathing in the pain clinic. Pain Med 2006;7(4):363–4.
[8] Collett BJ. Opioid tolerance: the clinical perspective. Br J Anaesth 1998;81:58–68.
[9] Portenoy RK. Opioid therapy for chronic nonmalignant pain: a review of critical issues. J Pain Symptom Manage 1996;11:203–17.
[10] Portenoy RK. Opioid therapy for chronic nonmalignant pain. Pain Res Manage 1996;1: 17–28.
[11] Urban BJ, France RD, Steinberger EK, et al. Long-term use of narcotic/antidepressant medication in the management of phantom limb pain. Pain 1986;24:191–6.
[12] Zenz M, Strumpf M, Tryba M. Long-term oral opioid therapy in patients with chronic nonmalignant pain. J Pain Symptom Manage 1992;7:69–77.
[13] Joint Commission on the Accreditation of Healthcare Organizations. Patient rights and organization ethics. Referenced from the comprehensive accreditation manual for hospitals, update 3, 1999. Available at: http://www.jointcommission.org. Accessed September 2006.
[14] Max MB, Payne R, Edwards WT, et al. Principles of analgesic use in the treatment of acute pain and cancer pain. 4th ed. Glenview, IL: American Pain Society; 1999.
[15] Katz N. The impact of pain management on quality of life. J Pain Symptom Manage 2002; 24(suppl 1):S38–47.
[16] Friedman R, Li V, Mehrotra D. Treating pain patients at risk: evaluation of a screening tool in opioid-treated pain patients with and without addiction. Pain Med 2003;4(2):182–5.
[17] Gavin DR, Ross HE, Skinner HA. Diagnostic validity of the drug abuse screening test in the assessment of DSM-III drug disorders. Br J Addict 1989;84(3):301–7.
[18] Butler SF, Budman SH, Fernandez K, et al. Validation of a screener and opioid assessment measure for patients with chronic pain. Pain 2004;112(1–2):65–75.
[19] Webster LR, Webster RM. Predicting aberrant behaviors in opioid-treated patients: preliminary validation of the Opioid Risk Tool. Pain Med 2005;6(6):432–42.
[20] Wincent A, Linden Y, Arner S. Pain questionnaires in the analysis of long lasting (chronic) pain conditions. Eur J Pain 2003;7:311–21.
[21] Clark JD. Chronic pain prevalence and analgesic prescribing in a general medical population. J Pain Symptom Manage 2002;23:131–7.

[22] Solomon DH, Schaffer JL, Katz JN, et al. Can history and physical examination be used as markers of quality? An analysis of the initial visit note in musculoskeletal care. Med Care 2000;38:383–91.

[23] Rhodes DJ, Koshy RC, Waterfield WC, et al. Feasibility of quantitative pain assessment in outpatient oncology practice. J Clin Oncol 2001;19:501–8.

[24] Passik SD, Schreiber J, Kirsh KL, et al. A chart review of the ordering and documentation of urine toxicology screens in a cancer center: do they influence patient management? J Pain Symptom Manage 2000;19:40–4.

[25] Passik SD, Weinreb HJ. Managing chronic nonmalignant pain: overcoming obstacles to the use of opioids. Adv Ther 2000;17:70–83.

[26] Passik SD, Kirsh KL, Whitcomb LA, et al. A new tool to assess and document pain outcomes in chronic pain patients receiving opioid therapy. Clin Ther 2004;26(4):552–61.

[27] Passik SD, Kirsh KL, Whitcomb LA, et al. Monitoring outcomes during long-term opioid therapy for non-cancer pain: results with the pain assessment and documentation tool. Journal of Opioid Management 2005;1(5):257–66.

[28] Daut R, Cleeland C, Flannery R. Development of the Wisconsin Brief Pain Questionnaire to assess pain in cancer and other diseases. Pain 1983;17:197–210.

[29] Cleeland CS, Ryan KM. Pain assessment: global use of the Brief Pain Inventory. Ann Acad Med Singapore 1994;23:129–38.

[30] Melzack R. The McGill Pain Questionnaire: major properties and scoring methods. Pain 1975;1:277–99.

[31] McCarberg BH, Barkin RL. Long-acting opioids for chronic pain: pharmacotherapeutic opportunities to enhance compliance, quality of life, and analgesia. Am J Ther 2001;8:181–6.

[32] Kalso E, Edwards JE, Moore RA, et al. Opioids in chronic non-cancer pain: systematic review of efficacy and safety. Pain 2004;112:372–80.

[33] Smith HS. The Numerical Opioid Side Effect (NOSE). Assessment tool. Journal of Cancer Pain and Symptom Palliation 2005;1:3–6.

[34] Turk DC, Dworkin RH, Allen RR, et al. Core outcome domains for chronic pain clinical trials: IMMPACT recommendations. Pain 2003;106:337–45.

[35] Smith HS. Translational analgesia and the translational analgesic score. Journal of Cancer Pain and Symptom Palliation 2005;1:15–9.

[36] Rogers WH, Wittink H, Wagner A, et al. Assessing individual outcomes during outpatient multidisciplinary chronic pain treatment by means of an augmented SF-36. Pain Med 2000;1:44–54.

[37] Rogers WH, Wittink H, Ashburn MA, et al. Using the "TOPS," an outcome instrument for multidisciplinary outpatient pain treatment. Pain Med 2000;1:55–67.

[38] Ware JE Jr, Sherbourne CD, The MOS. 36-item short-form health survey (SF-36). I. Conceptual Framework and Item Selection. Med Care 1992;30:473–83.

[39] Kerns R, Turk D, Rudy T. The West Haven-Yale Multidimensional Pain Inventory (WHYMPI). Pain 1985;23:345–6.

[40] Fairbanks J, Couper J, Davies J, et al. The Oswestry low back pain disability questionnaire. Physiotherapy 1980;66:271–3.

[41] Tarlor A, Ware J Jr, Greenfield S, et al. The Medical Outcomes Study: an application of methods for monitoring the results of medical care. JAMA 1989;262:925–30.

[42] Ruta DA, Garratt AM, Leng M, et al. A new approach to quality of life: the patient-generated index. Med Care 1994;32:1109–26.

[43] Smith HS. Perspectives in persistent noncancer pain. Journal of Cancer Pain and Symptom Palliation 2005c;1:31–2.

[44] Rome JD, Townsend CP, Bruce BK, et al. Chronic noncancer pain rehabilitation with opioid withdrawal: comparison of treatment outcomes based on opioid use status at admission. Mayo Clin Proc 2004;79:759–68.

[45] Holtman JR, Wala EP. Characterization of morphine-induced hyperalgesia in male and female rats. Pain 2005;114:62–70.

[46] Ruscheweyh R, Sand Kuhler J. Opioids and central sensitization: II. Induction and reversal of hyperalgesia. Eur J Pain 2005;9:149–52.

[47] Smith H, Audette J, Witkower A. Assessing analgesic therapeutic outcomes. In: Smith H, editor. Drugs for pain. Philadelphia (PA): H. Hanley and Belfus; 2003. p. 499–508.

[48] Smith HS, Audette J, Witkower A. Playing It "SAFE". Journal of Cancer Pain and Symptom Palliation 2005;1:3–10.

ELSEVIER
SAUNDERS

THE MEDICAL
CLINICS
OF NORTH AMERICA

Med Clin N Am 91 (2007) 229–239

Myofascial Trigger Points

Elizabeth Demers Lavelle, MD[a],
William Lavelle, MD[b],*, Howard S. Smith, MD, FACP[a]

[a]Department of Anesthesiology, Albany Medical Center, 43 New Scotland Avenue,
Albany, NY 12208, USA
[b]Department of Orthopaedic Surgery, 1367 Washington Avenue, Albany Medical Center,
Albany, NY 12206, USA

A myofascial trigger point is a hyperirritable point in skeletal muscle that is associated with a hypersensitive palpable nodule [1]. Approximately 23 million Americans have chronic disorders of the musculoskeletal system [2]. Painful conditions of the musculoskeletal system, including myofascial pain syndrome, constitute some of the most important chronic problems that are encountered in a clinical practice.

Definitions

Myofascial pain syndrome is defined as sensory, motor, and autonomic symptoms that are caused by myofascial trigger points. The sensory disturbances that are produced are dysesthesias, hyperalgesia, and referred pain. Coryza, lacrimation, salivation, changes in skin temperature, sweating, piloerection, proprioceptive disturbances, and erythema of the overlying skin are autonomic manifestations of myofascial pain.

Travell and Simons [1] defined the myofascial trigger point as "a hyper-irritable spot, usually within a taut band of skeletal muscle or in the muscle fascia which is painful on compression and can give rise to characteristic referred pain, motor dysfunction, and autonomic phenomena" [1]. When the trigger point is pressed, pain is caused and produces effects at a target, the zone of reference, or referral zone [3,4]. This area of referred pain is the feature that differentiates myofascial pain syndrome from fibromyalgia. This pain is reproduced reliably on palpation of the trigger point, despite the fact that it is remote from its source of origin. This referred pain rarely

---

* Corresponding author.
E-mail address: lavellwf@yahoo.com (W. Lavelle).

doi:10.1016/j.mcna.2006.12.004   *medical.theclinics.com*

coincides with dermatologic or neuronal distributions, but follows a consistent pattern [5].

Etiology

Trigger points may develop after an initial injury to muscle fibers. This injury may include a noticeable traumatic event or repetitive microtrauma to the muscles. The trigger point causes pain and stress in the muscle or muscle fiber. As the stress increases, the muscles become fatigued and more susceptible to activation of additional trigger points. When predisposing factors combine with a triggering stress event, activation of a trigger point occurs. This theory is known as the "injury pool theory" [1].

Pathophysiology

There is no pathologic or laboratory test for identifying trigger points. Therefore, much of the pathophysiologic research on trigger points has been directed toward verifying common theories of their formation. Fig. 1 provides an example of the theory behind the formation of myofascial trigger points.

The local twitch response (LTR) has been described as a characteristic response of myofascial trigger points. LTR is a brisk contraction of the muscle fibers in and around the taut band elicited by snapping palpation or rapid insertion of a needle into the myofascial trigger point [6]. The sensitive

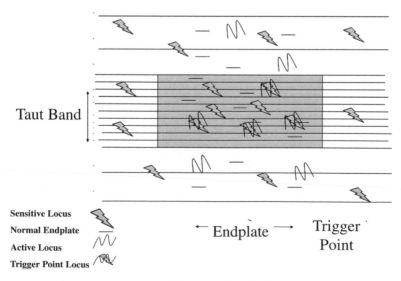

Fig. 1. Myofascial trigger point loci.

site where an LTR is found has been termed the "sensitive locus." Based on observations during successful trigger point injections, a model with multiple sensitive loci in a trigger point region was proposed [6]. In a recent histologic study, the sensitive loci correlated with sensory receptors [7,8].

In a study by Hubbard and Berkoff, spontaneous electrical activity was demonstrated at sites in a trigger point region, whereas similar activity was not found at adjacent nontender sites [6]. The site where the spontaneous electrical activity is recorded is termed the "active locus." To elicit and record spontaneous electrical activity, high-sensitivity recording and a gentle insertion technique into the trigger point must be used [6]. The waveforms of the spontaneous electrical activity correspond closely to previously published reports of motor endplate noise [9,10]. Therefore, the spontaneous electrical activity likely is one type of endplate potential, and the active loci probably are related closely to motor endplates.

It was hypothesized that a myofascial trigger point locus is formed when a sensitive locus, the nociceptor, and an active locus—the motor endplate—coincide. It is possible that sensitive loci are distributed widely throughout the entire muscle, but are concentrated in the trigger point region. This explains the finding of elicitation of referred pain when "normal" muscle tissue is needled or high pressure is applied (Fig. 2).

Diagnosis

The diagnosis of myofascial pain is best made through a careful analysis of the history of pain along with a consistent physical examination [11]. The diagnosis of myofascial pain syndrome, as defined by Simons and colleagues [12], relies on eight clinical characteristics (Box 1). Identification of the pain distribution is one of the most critical elements in identifying and treating myofascial pain. The physician should ask the patient to identify the most intense area of pain using a single finger. There also is an associated consistent and characteristic referred pain pattern on palpation of this trigger point. Often, this referred pain is not located in the immediate vicinity of the trigger point, but is found commonly in predictable patterns. These patterns are described clearly in *Travell and Simon's Myofascial Pain and Dysfunction: The Trigger Point Manual* [12]. Pain can be projected in a peripheral referral pattern, a central referral pattern, or a local pain pattern (Fig. 3). When a hyperintense area of pain is identified, its area of referred pain should be identified [4].

The palpable band is considered critical in the identification of the trigger point. Three methods have been identified for trigger point palpation: flat palpation, pincer palpation, and deep palpation. Flat palpation refers to sliding a fingertip across the muscle fibers of the affected muscle group. The skin is pushed to one side, and the finger is drawn across the muscle fibers. This process is repeated with the skin pushed to the other side. A taut band may be felt passing under the physician's finger. Snapping palpation,

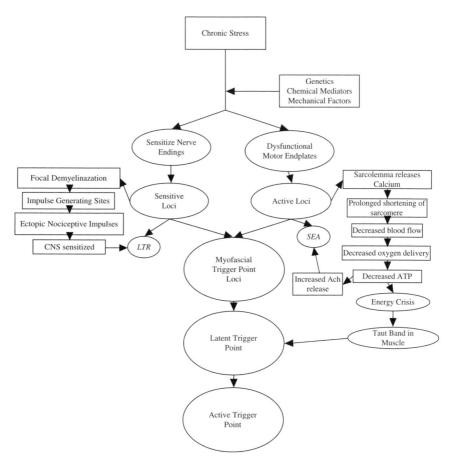

Fig. 2. Pathophysiology of myofascial trigger points. Ach, acetylcholine; CNS, central nervous system; LTR, local twitch response; SEA, spontaneous electrical activity.

like plucking of a violin, is used to identify the specific trigger point. Pincer palpation is a method that involves firmly grasping the muscle between the thumb and forefinger. The fibers are pressed between the fingers in a rolling manner while attempting to locate a taut band. Deep palpation may be used to find a trigger point that is obscured by superficial tissue. The fingertip is placed over the muscle attachment of the area suspected of housing the trigger point. When the patient's symptoms are reproduced by pressing in one specific direction, a trigger point may be presumed to be located [2].

Several devices have been developed to assist in the location of a myofascial trigger point. Fisher [13] developed a pressure threshold measuring gauge to assist in the diagnosis and location of the myofascial trigger point. It is a hand-held device calibrated in kg/cm^2. Pressure is increased gradually and evenly until the patient reports discomfort. The pressure measurement is then recorded. Contralateral pressure measurements are taken to establish

---

Box 1. Clinical characteristics of myofascial pain syndrome

Onset description and immediate cause of the pain
Pain distribution pattern
Restricted range of motion with increased sensitivity to
   stretching
Weakened muscle due to pain with no muscular atrophy
Compression causing pain similar to the patient's chief complaint
A palpable taut band of muscle correlating with the patient's
   trigger point
LTR elicited by snapping palpation or rapid insertion of a needle
Reproduction of the referred pain with mechanical stimulation of
   the trigger point

---

relative sensitivity of the point in question; a difference of 2 kg/cm^2 is considered an abnormal reading [14]. An electromyogram (EMG) also may assist in the diagnosis of the trigger point [15,16]. When the active locus is entered, the peak amplitudes often are off the scale of the EMG monitor. Although this method may seem to be useful scientifically, significant clinical results have not been found.

Noninvasive techniques for management

Spray (freeze) and stretch

Travell and Simons [1] advocated passive stretching of the affected muscle after application of sprayed vapocoolant to be the "single most effective treatment" for trigger point pain. The proper technique depends on patient education, cooperation, compliance, and preparation. The patient should be

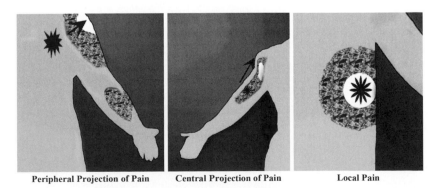

Peripheral Projection of Pain   Central Projection of Pain   Local Pain

Fig. 3. Trigger points and their reference zones.

positioned comfortably, ensuring that the trigger point area is well supported and under minimal tension. Position should place one end of the
muscle with the trigger point zone securely anchored. The patient should
be marked after careful diagnosis of the trigger point region, and the reference zone should be noted. The skin overlying the trigger point should be
anesthetized with a vapocoolant spray (ethyl chloride or dichlorodifluoro-
methane-trichloromonofluoromethane) over the entire length of the muscle
[12]. This spray should be applied from the trigger point toward the reference zone until the entire length of the muscle has been covered. The vapocoolant should be directed at a 30° angle to the skin. Immediately after the
first vapocoolant spray pass, passive pressure should be applied to the other
end of the muscle, resulting in a stretch. Multiple slow passes of spray over
the entire width of the muscle should be performed while maintaining the
passive muscle stretch. This procedure is repeated until full range of motion
of the muscle group is reached, with a maximum of three repetitions before
rewarming the area with moist heat. Care must be taken to avoid prolonged
exposure to the vapocoolant spray, assuring that each spray pass lasts less
than 6 seconds. Patients must be warned not to overstretch muscles after
a therapy session.

Physical therapy

Some of the best measures to relieve cyclic myofascial pain involve the
identification of perpetuating factors. Physical therapists assist patients in
the determination of predisposing activities. With routine follow-up, they
are often able to correct elements of poor posture and body mechanics [1].

Transcutaneous electrical stimulation

Transcutaneous electrical stimulation (TENS) is used commonly as adjuvant therapy in chronic and acute pain management. Placement of the
TENS electrode is an empiric process and may involve placement at trigger
point sites or along zones of referred pain [17].

Ultrasound

Ultrasound may be used as an adjunctive means of treatment. Ultrasound transmits vibration energy at the molecular level; approximately
50% reaches a depth of 5 mm.

Massage

Massage was advocated by Simons and colleagues [12]. Their technique
was described as a "deep stroking" or "stripping" massage. The patient is
positioned comfortably to allow the muscle group being treated to be
lengthened and relaxed as much as possible.

Ischemic compression therapy

The term "ischemic compression therapy" refers to the belief that the application of pressure to a trigger point produces ischemia that ablates the trigger point. Pressure is applied to the point with increasing resistance and maintained until the physician feels a relief of tension. The patient may feel mild discomfort, but should not experience profound pain. The process is repeated for each band of taut muscle encountered [12].

Invasive techniques for management

Trigger point injection remains the treatment with the most scientific evidence and investigation for support. Typically, it is advocated for trigger points that have failed noninvasive means for treatment. Injections are highly dependent of the clinician's skill to localize the active trigger point with a small needle.

Various injected substances have been investigated. These include local anesthetics, botulism toxin, sterile water, sterile saline, and dry needling. One common finding with these techniques is that, at least anecdotally, the duration of pain relief following the procedure outlasts the duration of action of the injected medication.

The universal technique for injection

The patient should be positioned in a recumbent position for the prevention of syncope, assistance in patient relaxation, and decreased muscle tension. The trigger point must then be identified correctly. The palpable band is considered critical in the identification of the trigger point. This can be done with any of the three methods described above. The trigger point should be marked clearly. Then, the skin is prepared in a sterile fashion. Various physicians use different skin preparations for their local procedures. One common skin preparation technique is to cleanse the skin with a topical alcohol solution followed by preparation with povidone-iodine [12]. A 22-gauge 1.5-inch needle is recommended for most superficial trigger points. Deeper muscles may be reached using a 21-gauge 2-inch or 2.5-inch needle. The needle should never be inserted to the hub because this is the weakest point on the needle [18].

Once the skin is prepared and the trigger point is identified, the overlying skin is grasped between the thumb and index finger or between the index and middle finger. The needle is inserted approximately 1 to 1.5 cm away from the trigger point to facilitate the advancement of the needle into the trigger point at a 30° angle. The grasping fingers isolate the taut band and prevent it from rolling out of the trajectory of the needle. A "fast-in, fast-out" technique should be used to elicit an LTR. This local twitch was shown to predict the effectiveness of the trigger point injection [19]. After entering the trigger point, the needle should be aspirated to ensure that the lumen of a local blood vessel has not been violated. If the physician chooses to inject an agent, a small volume should be injected at this time. The needle may be withdrawn to the level of the skin without exiting, and it should be redirected to the trigger point repeating the process. The process of entering the trigger point and eliciting LTRs should proceed, attempting to contact as many sensitive loci as possible (Fig. 4).

An integral part of trigger point therapy is postprocedural stretching. After trigger point injection, the muscle group that was injected should undergo a full active stretch.

Complications of trigger point injections

As with the introduction of any foreign body through the skin, the risk for skin or soft tissue infection is a possibility. Injection over an area of infected skin is contraindicated. The physician should never aim the needle at an intercostal space to avoid the complication of a pneumothorax. Hematoma formation following a trigger point injection can be minimized with proper injection technique and holding pressure over the surrounding soft tissue after withdrawal of the needle [12,20].

Medications for injection

Local anesthetics

Local anesthetics are the substances that have been investigated most frequently for the treatment of myofascial trigger points. Local anesthetic injections were shown to improve measures on a pain scale, range of motion,

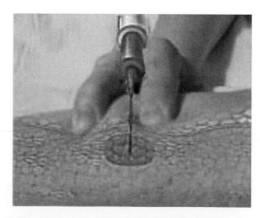

Fig. 4. Injection technique. The trigger point is positioned between two fingers to prevent the sliding of the trigger point during injection. The fingers are pressed downward and apart to maintain pressure and ensure hemostasis.

and algometry pressure thresholds. The volume of local anesthetic injected also has been investigated, and small volumes are considered the most effective. Typically, less than 1 mL of local agent should be injected in a highly controlled manner. The primary use for a local anesthetic is to prevent local soreness. Procaine is selected often because it is selective for small, unmyelinated fibers that control pain perception rather than motor control. Lidocaine is a common substitute for procaine, but no experimental comparisons are available in the literature [12,21].

Corticosteroids

Local steroid injections offer the potential advantage of control of local inflammatory response; however, the theory that a trigger point is due to a local energy crisis does not support their clinical use. Steroids are used commonly by the orthopedic surgeon and rheumatologist to treat local conditions, such as trigger finger and tennis elbow. They carry the added dangers of local myotoxicity, subcutaneous tissue damage, and skin discoloration [12].

Botulinum toxin

Localized injection of a small amount of commercially prepared botulism toxin A relaxes an overactive muscle by blocking the release of acetylcholine. This essentially denervates the muscle until new synaptic contacts can be established. When injecting botulism toxin, the physician should remember that the toxin does not discriminate between trigger points and normal motor endplates. The physician should be careful to localize the trigger point before injection [22,23].

Dry needling

Dry needling involves multiple advances of a needle into the muscle at the region of the trigger point. Much like any injection technique, the physician should aim to elicit an LTR, reproduction of the patient's symptomatology, and relief of muscle tension [7,24].

Summary

Myofascial pain syndromes are a widely recognized phenomenon among physicians and represent a common pain disorder in the American population. A myofascial trigger point is "a hyperirritable spot, usually within a taut band of skeletal muscle or in the muscle fascia. The spot is painful on compression and can give rise to characteristic referred pain, motor dysfunction, and autonomic phenomena" [1]. Many treatment strategies, both invasive and noninvasive, have been recognized for myofascial trigger points.

References

[1] Travell JG, Simons DG. Myofascial pain and dysfunction: the trigger point manual. Baltimore (MD): Williams and Wilkins; 1983.

[2] Imamura ST, Fischer AA, Imamura M, et al. Pain management using myofascial approach when other treatment failed. Physical Medicine & Rehabilitation Clinics of North America 1997;8(1):179–96.

[3] Maigne J, Maigne R. Trigger point of the posterior iliac crest: painful iliolumbar ligament insertion or cutaneous dorsal ramus pain? An anatomic study. Arch Phys Med Rehabil 1991;72(9):734–7.

[4] Sola A, Bonica J. Myofascial pain syndromes. In: Bonica J, Loeser J, Chapman S, et al, editors. The management of pain. Baltimore (MD): Lippincott Williams & Wilkins; 1996. p. 352–67.

[5] Long S, Kephart W. Myofascial pain syndrome. In: Ashburn M, Rice L, editors. The management of pain. New York: Churchill Livingstone, Inc.; 1998. p. 299–321.

[6] Simons D. Single-muscle myofascial pain syndromes. In: Tollison CD, Satterthwaite CD, Tollison J, editors. Handbook of pain management. 2nd edition. Baltimore (MD): Williams & Wilkins; 1994. p. 539–55.

[7] Hong C-Z. Trigger point injection: dry needling vs. lidocaine injection. Am J Phys Med Rehabil 1994;73:156–63.

[8] Hong C-Z, Chen J-T, Chen S-M, et al. Histological findings of responsive loci in a myofascial trigger spot of rabbit skeletal muscle fibers from where localized twitch responses could be elicited [abstract]. Arch Phys Med Rehabil 1996;77:962.

[9] Simons DG. Do endplate noise and spikes arise from normal motor endplates? Am J Phys Med Rehabil 2001;80:134–40.

[10] Simons DG, Hong C-Z, Simons LS. Endplate potentials are common to midfiber myofascial trigger points. Am J Phys Med Rehabil 2002;81:212–22.

[11] Graff-Radford S. Myofascial pain: diagnosis and management. Curr Pain Headache Rep 2004;8:463–7.

[12] Simons DG, Travell JG, Simons LS. Travell and Simon's myofascial pain and dysfunction: the trigger point manual. 2nd edition. Baltimore (MD): Williams and Wilkins; 1998.

[13] Fischer AA. Pressure threshold meter: its use for quantification of tender points. Arch Phys Med Rehabil 1986;67:836.

[14] Hong C-Z, Chen Y-N, Twehous D, et al. Pressure threshold for referred pain by compression on the trigger point and adjacent areas. Journal of Musculoskeletal Pain 1996;4: 61–79.

[15] Hubbard D, Berkhoff G. Myofascial trigger points show spontaneous needle EMG activity. Spine 1993;18:1803–7.

[16] Simons DG, Hong C-Z, Simons LS. Prevalence of spontaneous electrical activity at trigger spots and at control sites in rabbit skeletal muscle. Journal of Musculoskeletal Pain 1995;3: 35–48.

[17] Graff-Redford SB, Reeves JL, Baker RL, et al. Effects of transcutaneous electrical nerve stimulation on myofascial pain and trigger point sensitivity. Pain 1989;37:1–5.

[18] Ruane J. Identifying and injecting myofascial trigger points. Phys Sportsmed 2001;29(12): 49–53.

[19] Hong C-Z, Simons DG. Response to standard treatment for pectoralis minor myofascial pain syndrome after whiplash. Journal of Musculoskeletal Pain 1993;1:89–131.

[20] Hong C-Z, Simons D. Pathophysiologic and electrophysiologic mechanisms of myofascial trigger points. Arch Phys Med Rehabil 1998;79:863–72.

[21] Hubbard D. Chronic and recurrent muscle pain: pathophysiology and treatment, and review of pharmacologic studies. Journal of Musculoskeletal Pain 1996;4:123–43.

[22] Acquandro MA, Borodic GE. Treatment of myofascial pain with botulism toxin A. Anesthesiology 1994;80:705–6.
[23] Cheshire WP, Abashian SW, Mann JD. Botulism toxin in the treatment of myofascial pain syndrome. Pain 1994;59:65–9.
[24] Chen J, Chung K, Hou C, et al. Inhibitory effect of dry needling on the spontaneous electrical activity recorded from myofascial trigger points of rabbit skeletal muscle. Am J Phys Med Rehabil 2001;80:729–35.

THE MEDICAL
CLINICS
OF NORTH AMERICA

ELSEVIER
SAUNDERS

Med Clin N Am 91 (2007) 241–250

Intra-Articular Injections

William Lavelle, MD[a],*,
Elizabeth Demers Lavelle, MD[b], Lori Lavelle, DO[c]

[a]Department of Orthopaedic Surgery, Albany Medical Center, 1367 Washington Avenue,
Albany, NY 12206, USA
[b]Department of Anesthesiology, Albany Medical Center, 43 New Scotland Avenue,
Albany, NY 12208, USA
[c]Department of Rheumatology, Altoona Arthritis and Osteoporosis Center,
1125 Old Route 220N, Duncansville, PA 16635, USA

Intra-articular injections are one method that physicians may use to treat joint pain. Corticosteroids were the first substances to be injected commonly into the intra-articular space. In the 1950s, corticosteroids were found to lower indicators of the inflammatory response, including the interarticular leukocyte count [1,2]. The indications and effectiveness of intra-articular steroid injections have been debated since their introduction. More recently, viscosupplementation has gained popularity. Local anesthetics also have become common additions to intra-articular injections. Anesthesiologists and orthopedic surgeons have started to explore the use of intra-articular opiates for postoperative analgesia.

Injections for chronic joint pain

Steroid injections

Joint aspiration was described as early as the 1930s. The first intra-articular injectates, which yielded little benefit, were formalin and glycerin, lipodol, lactic acid, and petroleum jelly [3,4]. Hollander [5,6] attempted joint injections with hydrocortisone acetate and found that his patients had a much better clinical response in a series of more than 100,000 injections in 4000 patients. From the 1950s to the present, physicians have used corticosteroid injections routinely to treat joint pain.

Clinical efficacy has been shown for intra-articular injections of steroids in the treatment of rheumatoid arthritis. In a randomized study, patients

* Corresponding author.
E-mail address: lavellwf@yahoo.com (W. Lavelle).

who were treated with intra-articular injections demonstrated significantly better pain control and range of motion than did those who were treated with mini-pulse systemic steroids. Patient evaluation of disease activity, tender joint count, blood pressure, side effects, calls to the physician, and hospital visits were significantly better ($P < .05$) for those who were treated with intra-articular steroids [7].

Mechanism of action of intra-articular steroid injections

Steroids possess anti-inflammatory properties. On the cellular level, steroids are highly lipophilic and are believed to bind to the cell's nucleus. It is believed that steroids act by altering transcription. Intra-articular steroids seem to reduce the number of lymphocytes, macrophages, and mast cells [8,9]; this, in turn, reduces phagocytosis, lysosomal enzyme release, and the release of inflammatory mediators [1]. Inflammation is reduced, particularly through reductions in the release of interleukin-1, leukotrienes, and prostaglandins [10,11]. With the reduction of these inflammatory mediators, pain symptoms often are improved.

Because they are injected locally, intra-articular steroids avoid most of the systemic effects of oral steroids, including muscle weakness, skin thinning resulting in easy bruising, peptic ulceration, and aggravation of diabetes.

Skin preparation

Skin preparation is as individualized as that seen for surgical site preparation. In a survey of orthopedists and rheumatologists, approximately half used alcohol swabs and the other half used chlorhexidine or povidine-iodine. Less than 20% used sterile towels to isolate the injection site, and only 32.5% of respondents used sterile gloves [12]. The authors recommend preparation with alcohol followed by preparation with Betadine and the use of sterile gloves.

Choice of steroid

Based strictly on chemical structure, the duration of effect should be inversely proportional to the solubility of the steroid (Table 1). There have

Table 1
Steroid solubility

Steroid	Solubility (% wt/vol)
Hydrocortisone acetate	0.002
Methylprednisolone acetate	0.001
Prednisolone tebutate	0.001
Triamcinolone acetate	0.004
Triamcinolone hexacetonide	0.0002

been conflicting studies on the duration of action of various steroids. Little data exist touting the true efficacy of one agent over another. In most cases, the choice of steroid is related to the personal preference of the physician rather than true science. In a survey performed on members of the 1994 American College of Rheumatology, approximately one third favored methylprednisolone, one third favored triamcinolone hexacetonide, and one fifth favored triamcinolone acetonide [9,13].

Use of local anesthetic

At times, local anesthetics (eg, lidocaine) are combined with the steroid. Some physicians contend that the local agent dilutes the steroid crystals, but it is unclear whether this process has any impact on the effect of the steroid. Lidocaine may have a transient anti-inflammatory effect in and of itself [14,15].

Adverse reactions

The most obvious concern about intra-articular injections is infection; however, few orthopedists and rheumatologists have encountered a case of poststeroid septic arthritis [12]. Avoidance of this complication depends on strict adherence to sterile technique. Suspicion of an intra-articular infection or an overlying soft tissue infection contraindicates the injection of a joint with corticosteroid. Other contraindications include a local fracture of total joint. Recent reports found infection rates of between 1 in 3000 and 1 in 50,000 [12]. *Staphylococcus aureus* is the most common infecting organism [12,16].

Mild local reactions do occur after injection. Postinjection flares occurred in about 2% to 6% of patients and were believed to result from chemical synovitis in response to the injected crystals [17]. Facial flushing may be seen in up to 15% of patients, mostly in women [8]. Skin or fat atrophy may be observed at the actual site of needle entry [17]. There is some concern regarding the use of intra-articular steroid injections in the diabetic population. Transient increases in blood glucose may be seen in patients receiving corticosteroid injections; however, in a study of diabetic patients who received soft tissue injections of methylprednisolone acetate, there was no detectable effect on blood glucose levels in the 14 days after injection [18]. Intra-articular steroids also transiently affect the hypothalamic–pituitary–adrenal axis. These changes, which include a 21.5% reduction in serum cortisol levels, typically normalize within 3 days, although an episode of Cushing's syndrome was reported [19,20].

Joint destruction after repetitive injections is a common concern. Animal studies have been suggestive of damage to articular cartilage because of intra-articular steroid injections; however, there are no human data to corroborate this claim [10]. Because of fear of possible joint destruction, many physicians recommend 3 months between injections of the same joint [13,21].

Clinical trials

One of the largest clinical trials of intra-articular steroid injections was done in the 1950s by Hollander [5,6]. Hydrocortisone injections of 1034 knees with osteoarthritis revealed an 80% success rate. Since that time, a multitude of studies proved the excellent short-term pain relief (1–4 weeks) gained from injected corticosteroids [21]. Longer-term results were not proved in consecutive studies; however, the short-term pain relief may allow the patient to return to baseline function and improve one's ability to perform physical therapy [22,23].

An adjunct to the success of steroid treatment in the patient who has an effusion may be the aspiration of that effusion. Eighty-four patients who had osteoarthritis were randomized to receive triamcinolone hexacetonide or placebo. Patients who received the steroid reported a statistically significant improvement in pain, distance walked in 1 minute, and Health Assessment Questionnaire score. Among patients who were treated with steroids, those who had an effusion that was aspirated at the time of injection showed greater improvement ($P<.05$) [24]. Joint lavage similarly improved pain and function if performed at the time of steroid injection [25].

Hyaluronic acid

Intra-articular steroids are not the only materials that are injected intra-articularly in the treatment of osteoarthritis. A randomized, placebo-controlled study compared more than 100 patients who received hyaluronic acid, corticosteroid (methylprednisolone acetate), or isotonic saline. These injections were placed with the aid of ultrasound. Injections were administered at 14-day intervals, with each patient receiving three injections. Significant improvement was seen at 3 months in the population that was treated with corticosteroid compared with patients who were treated with saline ($P = .006$ at 14 days, $P = .006$ at 28 days, and $P = .58$ at 3 months), whereas improvement in the group that was treated with hyaluronic acid failed to reach statistical significance ($P = .069$ at 14 days, $P =.14$ at 28 days, and $P =.57$ at 3 months). Statistically, there was no significant difference between hyaluronic acid and corticosteroid at any time point ($P>.21$) [26].

Postoperative intra-articular analgesia

The analgesic effects of intra-articular agents in the postoperative period are controversial; however, their use is becoming more common in the outpatient orthopedic setting [27]. The use of peripheral blocks for extremity surgery requires greater skill in placement and has a potential for significant complications [27]. Arthroscopy has been described as a method for orthopedic improvement with decreased morbidity, but not one of decreased pain [28,29]. Poor pain control may prevent a procedure from being acceptable in an outpatient setting, therefore, postoperative analgesia becomes an important consideration for outpatient surgery centers. Intra-articular analgesia techniques are used most commonly for knee and shoulder surgery. With some debate, intra-articular administration of local agents has proven effective for knee arthroscopy [30–38]; however, pain control for the shoulder has proven a greater task. Severe pain scores have been reported for even the most minor shoulder procedures [39].

Local agents

Most anesthesiologists and orthopedic surgeons select bupivacaine because of its long duration of action. This does not preclude the use of other local agents. The literature on the use of intra-articular local anesthetics includes numerous studies, but it is difficult to interpret because of the use of confounding agents, such as intra-articular opiates, clonidine, and nonsteroidals. A large number of these studies also is flawed with regard to study design, data collection, and reporting. A systematic review of double-blind, randomized, controlled trials that compared intra-articular local with placebo or no intervention and found a statistically significant improved pain after intra-articular local in pain scores. Pain scores were significantly lower in the treatment group and the amount of supplemental analgesics requested was reduced by 10% to 50%. The presence of hemarthrosis, which can increase the level of pain and decrease the concentration of local agents, is another factor that may alter the activity of intra-articular local analgesia [37]. Although the data from this review seem to indicate that intra-articular local analgesia is only mildly effective, its use in the outpatient orthopedic setting is a popular and safe adjuvant [40].

A continuous infusion of intra-articular analgesia was examined. In a prospective randomized trial of 50 subjects who underwent acromioplasty and rotator cuff repair and received a multiorifice catheter placed in the subacromial space, no statistically significant difference in pain scores or patient-controlled analgesic use was detected [41].

Opiates

Opioid receptors have been discovered in the peripheral nervous system. Mu, delta, and kappa receptors were found on peripheral nerves [37,42]. The effectiveness of opiates in inflamed tissues has been explained by a disruption in the perineurium, allowing for easier access of opioids to neuronal receptors. This also may be associated with an unmasking or up-regulation of inactive opiate receptors [37,43]. It was proposed that the effects of intra-articular morphine might simply be due to systemic absorption; however, the plasma concentration achieved from an intra-articular injection would be far too low for a systemic effect to be observed [37]. Within the joint itself, the relative concentration is high.

Kalso and colleagues [44] reviewed 36 randomized controlled trials. Four of the six studies that compared opiates with placebo found greater efficacy for intra-articular morphine. Four of the six studies that compared intra-articular morphine with intravenous or intramuscular morphine showed greater efficacy for intra-articular morphine. Several dosages were used with varying effects in the literature reviewed. Specifically, the minimum dose tested (0.5 mg) did not show efficacy, but a dose of 1 mg did. No greater effect was found when a dose of 1 mg was compared with 2 mg [44,45].

In a review by Gupta and colleagues [46], a meta-analysis was completed on the pooled data of 19 prospective, placebo-controlled, randomized studies in which intra-articular morphine was used. Within these studies, visual analog scores were collected at the early phase (0–2 hours), the intermediate phase (2–6 hours), and the late phase (6–24 hours). This analysis concluded that although no clear dose-response effect was seen, a definite, but mild, analgesic effect was present.

Another recent review is a bit more skeptical. Rosseland and colleagues reviewed randomized controlled trials that involved the use of intra-articular morphine [29]. In the 43 publications included, some of which were included in the reviews by Kalso and colleagues [44] and Gupta and colleagues [46], 23 were believed to be of low scientific quality with poor randomization and blinding or unsound statistics. Thirteen were believed to have usable information; however, four of the positive outcomes were believed to be due to the uneven distribution of patients whose natural course was low postoperative pain. The only randomized control trial that Rosseland believed was adequate was negative [47].

Clonidine

Intra-articular clonidine also has been investigated. Clonidine is an α-agonist that was shown to prolong the duration of local anesthetics. In a controlled study, 40 patients who underwent knee arthroscopy were randomized to receive intra-articular clonidine in combination with 1 mg of morphine. Patients who received clonidine had significantly longer analgesia durations [37].

Many physicians who participate in outpatient orthopedic surgery recommend a multimodal approach consisting of intra-articular agents, including local analgesia, an opiate, and an adjunct (eg, clonidine) [37]. The specifics of

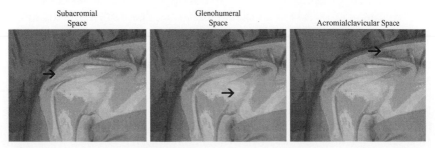

Fig. 1. Spaces in the shoulder that may be treated by an intra-articular injection.

Lateral Para patella
Portal

Medial Para patella
Portal

Superior Lateral
Portal

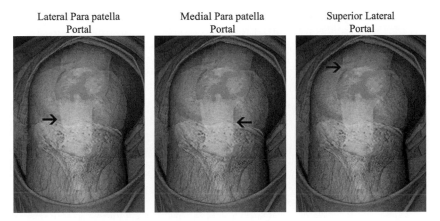

Fig. 2. Different approaches used to access the knee for an intra-articular injection.

the injectate are left to the individual. Local analgesia seems to be helpful early in the postoperative period (2-4 hours) to prevent a deleterious physiologic pain response. Intra-articular morphine may be more helpful in the hours afterward. In general, the use of pre-emptive and multimodal analgesia is important to abate postoperative pain, with an emphasis on minimizing systemic narcotic analgesia, which has the deleterious effects of respiratory depression, sedation, nausea, puritis, and delayed discharge [37].

Techniques to improve placement

Figs. 1 and 2 illustrate the anatomic locations for injections into the shoulder and knee. It is truly with repetition that the physician becomes facile with most intra-articular injections. Image guidance with the aid of ultrasound or fluoroscopy is a valuable tool to help access difficult joints, such as the hip. Fluoroscopy and a radiopaque tracer allow for documented delivery of an agent into a joint. Aspiration of synovial fluid before injection of a steroid is one method that may allow for improved accuracy. One study examined this question. A recent article assessed the accuracy of needle placement in the intra-articular space of the knee using three common knee joint portals. The investigators documented the location of the injected fluid by fluoroscopic imaging. They found far more success with a lateral midpatellar injection than with either of the other injection portals [47].

Summary

Intra-articular injections provide physicians with one modality to treat chronic or acute joint pain. Whatever method is chosen, careful attention to the anatomic landmarks and experience are critical to the successful placement of an intra-articular injection. Intra-articular steroid injections have been used for management of inflammatory joint diseases, such as arthritis. Occasionally, local anesthetics are injected in combination with the steroids. New studies found that intra-articular injections may be helpful for the management of postoperative pain, particularly with the use of opiates.

References

[1] Snibbe JC, Gambardella RA. Use of injections for osteoarthritis in joints and sports activity. Clin Sports Med 2005;24(1):83–91.
[2] Hollander JL, Brown EM Jr, Jessar RA, et al. Hydrocortisone and cortisone injected into arthritic joints; comparative effects of and use of hydrocortisone as a local antiarthritic agent. JAMA 1951;147(17):1629–35.
[3] Pemberton R. Arthritis and rheumatoid conditions. Their nature and treatment. Philadelphia: Lea and Febiger; 1935.
[4] Ropes MW, Bauer W. Synovial fluid changes in joint disease. Cambridge (MA): Harvard University Press; 1953.
[5] Hollander JL. Hydrocortisone and cortisone injected into arthritic joints. Comparative effects of and use of hydrocortisone as a local antiarthritic agent. JAMA 1951;147:1629.
[6] Hollander JL. Intrasynovial corticosteroid therapy: a decade of use. Bull Rheum Dis 1961; 11:239.
[7] Furtado RN, Oliveira LM, Natour J. Polyarticular corticosteroid injection versus systemic administration in treatment of rheumatoid arthritis patients: a randomized controlled study. J Rheumatol 2005;32(9):1691–8.
[8] Cole BJ, Schumacher HR Jr. Injectable corticosteroids in modern practice. J Am Acad Orthop Surg 2005;13(1):37–46.
[9] Centeno LM, Moore ME. Preferred intraarticular corticosteroids and associated practice: a survey of members of the American College of Rheumatology. Arthritis Care Res 1994; 7(3):151–5.
[10] Uthman I, Raynauld JP, Haraoui B. Intra-articular therapy in osteoarthritis. Postgrad Med J 2003;79(934):449–53.
[11] Wilder RL. Corticosteroids. In: Klippel JH, Cornelia WM, Wortmann RL, editors. Primer on rheumatic diseases. Atlanta (GA): Arthritis Foundation; 1997. p. 427–31.
[12] Charalambous CP, Tryfonidis M, Sadiq S, et al. Septic arthritis following intra-articular steroid injection of the knee–a survey of current practice regarding antiseptic technique used during intra-articular steroid injection of the knee. Clin Rheumatol 2003;22(6): 386–90.
[13] Rozental TD, Sculco TP. Intra-articular corticosteroids: an updated overview. Am J Orthop 2000;29(1):18–23.
[14] Schumacher HR Jr. Aspiration and injection therapies for joints. Arthritis Rheum 2003; 49(3):413–20.
[15] Paul H, Clayburne G, Schumacher HR. Lidocaine inhibits leukocyte migration and phagocytosis in monosodium urate crystal-induced synovitis in dogs. J Rheumatol 1983;10(3): 434–9.
[16] von Essen R, Savolainen HA. Bacterial infection following intra-articular injection. A brief review. Scand J Rheumatol 1989;18(1):7–12.
[17] Kumar N, Newman RJ. Complications of intra- and peri-articular steroid injections. Br J Gen Pract 1999;49(443):465–6.
[18] Slotkoff A, Clauw D, Nashel D. Effect of soft tissue corticosteroid injection on glucose control in diabetics. Arthritis Rheum 1994;37(Suppl 9):S347.
[19] Emkey RD, Lindsay R, Lyssy J, et al. The systemic effect of intraarticular administration of corticosteroid on markers of bone formation and bone resorption in patients with rheumatoid arthritis. Arthritis Rheum 1996;39(2):277–82.

[20] Roberts WN, Babcock EA, Breitbach SA, et al. Corticosteroid injection in rheumatoid arthritis does not increase rate of total joint arthroplasty. J Rheumatol 1996;23(6):1001–4.

[21] Chumacher HR, Chen LX. Injectable corticosteroids in treatment of arthritis of the knee. Am J Med 2005;118(11):1208–14.

[22] Godwin M, Dawes M. Intra-articular steroid injections for painful knees. Systematic review with meta-analysis. Can Fam Physician 2004;50:241–8.

[23] Arroll B, Goodyear-Smith F. Corticosteroid injections for painful shoulder: a meta-analysis. Br J Gen Pract 2005;55(512):224–8.

[24] Gaffney K, Ledingham J, Perry JD. Intra-articular triamcinolone hexacetonide in knee osteoarthritis: factors influencing the clinical response. Ann Rheum Dis 1995;54(5):379–81.

[25] Ravaud P, Moulinier L, Giraudeau B, et al. Effects of joint lavage and steroid injection in patients with osteoarthritis of the knee: results of a multicenter, randomized, controlled trial. Arthritis Rheum 1999;42(3):475–82.

[26] Qvistgaard E, Christensen R, Torp-Pedersen S, et al. Intra-articular treatment of hip osteoarthritis: a randomized trial of hyaluronic acid, corticosteroid, and isotonic saline. Osteoarthritis Cartilage 2006;14(2):163–70.

[27] Savoie FH, Field LD, Jenkins RN, et al. The pain control infusion pump for postoperative pain control in shoulder surgery. Arthroscopy 2000;16(4):339–42.

[28] Rawal N. Incisional and intra-articular infusions. Best Pract Res Clin Anaesthesiol 2002; 16(2):321–43.

[29] Rosseland LA, Helgesen KG, Breivik H, et al. Moderate-to-severe pain after knee arthroscopy is relieved by intraarticular saline: a randomized controlled trial. Anesth Analg 2004; 98(6):1546–51.

[30] Geutjens G, Hambidge JE. Analgesic effects of intraarticular bupivacaine after day-case arthroscopy. Arthroscopy 1994;10(3):299–300.

[31] Morrow BC, Milligan KR, Murthy BV. Analgesia following day-case knee arthroscopy–the effect of piroxicam with or without bupivacaine infiltration. Anaesthesia 1995;50(5):461–3.

[32] Vranken JH, Vissers K, de Jongh R, et al. Intraarticular sufentanil administration facilitates recovery after day-case knee arthroscopy. Anesth Analg 2001;92:625–8.

[33] Henderson RC, Campion ER, DeMasi RA, et al. Postarthroscopy analgesia with bupivacaine. A prospective, randomized, blinded evaluation. Am J Sports Med 1990;18(6):614–7.

[34] Osborne D, Keene G. Pain relief after arthroscopic surgery of the knee: a prospective, randomized, and blinded assessment of bupivacaine and bupivacaine with adrenaline. Arthroscopy 1993;9(2):177–80.

[35] Aasbo V, Raeder JC, Grogaard B, et al. No additional analgesic effect of intra-articular morphine or bupivacaine compared with placebo after elective knee arthroscopy. Acta Anaesthesiol Scand 1996;40(5):585–8.

[36] Highgenboten CL, Jackson AW, Meske NB. Arthroscopy of the knee. Ten-day pain profiles and corticosteroids. Am J Sports Med 1993;21(4):503–6.

[37] Reuben SS, Sklar J. Pain management in patients who undergo outpatient arthroscopic surgery of the knee. J Bone Joint Surg Am 2000;82-A(12):1754–66.

[38] Dye SF, Vaupel GL, Dye CC. Conscious neurosensory mapping of the internal structures of the human knee without intraarticular anesthesia. Am J Sports Med 1998;26(6):773–7.

[39] Ritchie ED, Tong D, Chung F, et al. Suprascapular nerve block for postoperative pain relief in arthroscopic shoulder surgery: a new modality? Anesth Analg 1997;84(6):1306–12.

[40] Meinig RP, Holtgrewe JL, Wiedel JD, et al. Plasma bupivacaine levels following single dose intraarticular instillation for arthroscopy. Am J Sports Med 1988;16(3):295–300.

[41] Boss AP, Maurer T, Seiler S, et al. Continuous subacromial bupivacaine infusion for postoperative analgesia after open acromioplasty and rotator cuff repair: preliminary results. J Shoulder Elbow Surg 2004;13(6):630–4.

[42] Stein C, Millan MJ, Shippenberg TS, et al. Peripheral opioid receptors mediating antinociception in inflammation. Evidence for involvement of mu, delta and kappa receptors. J Pharmacol Exp Ther 1989;248(3):1269–75.

[43] Stein C, Yassouridis A. Peripheral morphine analgesia. Pain 1997;71(2):119–21.

[44] Kalso E, Tramer MR, Carroll D, et al. Pain relief from intra-articular morphine after knee surgery: a qualitative systematic review. Pain 1997;71(2):127–34.

[45] Allen GC, St Amand MA, Lui AC, et al. Postarthroscopy analgesia with intraarticular bupivacaine/morphine. A randomized clinical trial. Anesthesiology 1993;79(3):475–80.

[46] Gupta A, Bodin L, Holmstrom B, et al. A systematic review of the peripheral analgesic effects of intraarticular morphine. Anesth Analg 2001;93(3):761–70.

[47] Jackson DW, Evans NA, Thomas BM. Accuracy of needle placement into the intra-articular space of the knee. J Bone Joint Surg Am 2002;84-A(9):1522–7.

ELSEVIER
SAUNDERS

Med Clin N Am 91 (2007) 251–270

THE MEDICAL
CLINICS
OF NORTH AMERICA

Intrathecal Analgesia

Steven P. Cohen, MD[a,b,*], Anthony Dragovich, MD[b]

[a]Pain Management Division, Department of Anesthesiology,
Johns Hopkins School of Medicine, 550 North Broadway, Suite 301,
Baltimore, MD 21205, USA
[b]Department of Surgery, Walter Reed Army Medical Center, Anesthesia Service,
6900 Georgia Avenue, NW, Washington, DC 20307, USA

The discovery of opioid receptors in neural tissue in the early 1970s [1,2] provided the impetus for the treatment of pain by injecting analgesic medications directly into the spinal canal, first in experimental animals [3], then in cancer patients [4]. In many respects the treatment of cancer pain with intrathecal (IT) opioids is an ideal scenario, given the high incidence of severe pain in terminal patients [5], the likelihood of developing dose-limiting side effects when oral opioids are used to treat pain, and concerns regarding issues of tolerance, dependence, and addiction. Previous reviews have demonstrated excellent outcomes using IT analgesia in patients with malignancies, although for financial reasons some experts recommend tunneled epidural catheters in lieu of implantable infusion devices in patients with life expectancies under 3 months [6].

The main controversy surrounding spinal analgesia is whether it is effective in the long term for nonmalignant pain. Current issues that permeate the ongoing debate on opioid use for noncancer pain include evidence that opioid-induced hyperalgesia accounts for a significant component of narcotic tolerance; literature suggesting that whereas opioids do provide short-term pain relief, their long-term ability to attenuate pain and improve function are less convincing; and higher estimates from better studies on the incidence of addiction in chronic pain patients [7–9].

The opinions or assertions contained herein are the private views of the authors and are not to be construed as official or as reflecting the views of the Department of the Army or the Department of Defense.

Funded in part by the John P. Murtha Neuroscience and Pain Institute, Johnstown, PA, and the U.S. Department of Defense.

* Corresponding author.

E-mail address: scohen40@jhmi.edu (S.P. Cohen).

We believe that implantable IT pumps have a place in the treatment of chronic, nonmalignant pain, albeit with certain caveats. Similar to prescribing oral and parenteral opioids, patients should be screened for signs of abuse, aberrant behavior, and psychological conditions that might predispose patients to failure before embarking on an IT trial. Although IT pumps are less prone to abuse than systemic opioids and carry almost no risk of diversion, the dependent relationship established by the implantation of an IT infusion device makes risk stratification just as essential [10]. A recent report by Kittelberger and colleagues [11] described a patient with failed back surgery syndrome (FBSS) who self-extracted hydromorphone from his pump.

Consideration should also be given to the likelihood of treatment success. Patients who have not acquiesced to trials with less invasive treatments are probably poor candidates for IT therapy. Certain medical conditions are more amenable to IT therapy than others. For example, IT baclofen is well-documented to be an effective treatment for spasticity-related pain, and zicontide was demonstrated in a recent multicenter randomized, controlled study to be effective in AIDS [12]. For opioid therapy, there are studies that support treatment in herpes zoster, but little evidence for their use in fibromyalgia.

Finally, in patients who otherwise meet criteria for consideration of IT therapy, a trial with either IT or epidural medications is of paramount importance. This holds true irrespective of the intended analgesic medication(s). But short-term trials are not without drawbacks. Some limitations of IT trials include the lack of standardization regarding the types (combinations) and doses of medications administered, limited outcome measures, and the fact that while short-term trials may predict short- and intermediate-term pain relief, their ability to prognosticate long-term outcomes is less established. For long-term therapy, the main factors limiting success are the development of tolerance and side effects, neither of which can be accurately predicted with a short-term trial (Box 1).

Opioids

Opioid receptors are characterized into three subtypes: mu, delta, and kappa, all of which are G-protein complexes [13]. The analgesic and nonanalgesic effects of opioids are mediated pre- and postsynaptically. Opioid binding to presynaptic terminals results in inhibition of substance P and calcitonin gene-related peptide release through suppression of voltage-gated calcium channels [14]. Postsynaptically, opioids cause inhibition of adenyl cyclase and activation of inwardly rectifying potassium currents resulting in neuronal hyperpolarization [15].

The effects of opioids are determined by their affinity for endogenous receptors and their ability to reach those receptors. In general, there is

---

Box 1. Selection criteria for intrathecal pump placement

- Stable medical condition amenable to surgery
- Clear organic pain generator
- No psychological or sociological contraindication
- No familial contraindication such as severe codependent behavior
- Documented responsible behavior and stable social situation
- Good pain relief with oral or parenteral opioids
- Intolerable side effects from systemic opioid therapy
- Baseline neurological exam and psychological evaluation
- Failure of more conservative therapy including trials with nonopioid medications and nerve blocks
- Constant or almost constant pain requiring around-the-clock opioid therapy
- High degree of tolerance to opioids may limit effectiveness of intrathecal therapy
- No tumor encroachment of thecal sac in cancer patients
- Life expectancy > 3 months
- No practical issues that might interfere with device placement, maintenance, or assessment (eg, morbid obesity, severe cognitive impairment)
- Positive response to an intrathecal trial

---

a positive correlation between the degree of water solubility and both the spread of analgesia and side effects. Highly water-soluble opioids like morphine exhibit a greater degree of rostral spread when injected intrathecally, which may improve analgesia in conditions requiring higher spinal levels or more extensive coverage. Conversely, many of the most common (pruritis and vomiting) and feared (delayed respiratory depression) adverse effects of spinal opioids are a result of interactions with opioid receptors in the brain, and thus are more frequently encountered with hydrophilic drugs like morphine (Table 1).

There is increasing evidence that IT opioids are superior to oral delivery in malignant pain, especially when narcotic dosage is limited by side effects.

Table 1
Conversion ratios between commonly used opioid agonists

Opioid	Oral	Parenteral	Epidural	Intrathecal	Hydrophilicity
Morphine	300	200	10	1	High
Hydromorphone	60	20	2	0.2	Intermediate
Meperidine	3000	1000	100	10	Low
Fentanyl	—	1	0.1	0.01	Low
Sufentanil	—	0.1	0.01	0.001	Low

In a multicenter, randomized trial, Smith and colleagues [16] compared IT drug delivery to comprehensive medical management (CMM) in 200 cancer patients. The mean visual analogue scale (VAS) pain score in the IT group fell 52%, which favorably compared with the 39% decrease in the CMM group. Toxicity scores in the CMM group fell 17% versus 50% in pump patients. Although not considered a primary outcome measure, 6-month survival in the IT drug delivery group was 54% compared with 37% in CMM patients. Whereas the large majority of studies assessing IT opioids in cancer pain have demonstrated reduced pain and improved function and quality of life, not all have been uniformly positive. In a multicenter, prospective, open-label study, Rauck and colleagues [17] evaluated a patient-activated IT morphine delivery system in 119 cancer patients with either refractory pain or uncontrollable side effects. One-month postimplant, the mean numerical pain score decreased from 6.1 to 4.2 (31%), a difference that persisted for 13 months. A statistically significant reduction was also noted for toxicity and oral opioid requirements. However at the final 16-month follow-up, the difference between baseline and current pain scores was no longer significant.

The evidence supporting IT opioids in nonmalignant pain is less robust than for cancer pain. To some extent, this may be because of different pain mechanisms characterizing the two conditions. In cancer, between 75% and 90% of pain is either nociceptive or mixed nociceptive-neuropathic in origin [18,19]. In nonmalignant pain, the etiology is more variable. For the chronic nonmalignant conditions most amenable to spinal analgesia such as FBSS, neuropathic pain tends to play a significant role. Numerous preclinical [20] and clinical [21] studies have shown neuropathic pain to be less responsive to opioids than nociceptive pain.

Thimineur and colleagues [22] conducted a prospective study comparing outcomes for chronic nonmalignant pain in patients who received IT opioid therapy (n = 38) with patients who either failed their trial or refused pump implant (n = 31), and newly referred patients who were not offered IT therapy (n = 41). During the 3-year study, VAS pain scores, functional capacity, and mood scores improved significantly in the pump recipients, while they either declined or stayed the same in nonpump recipients. However, most IT patients continued to suffer from moderate to severe pain. The authors concluded that while patients with severe, refractory pain will likely improve with IT therapy, their overall pain and symptom severity will remain high. To summarize the existing studies evaluating IT opioids for noncancer pain, most show significant short- to intermediate-term improvement for both neuropathic and nociceptive pain, but rarely is pain completely eradicated, and improvement in other outcome parameters (eg, mood and functional capacity) is less impressive (Table 2).

The most frequent causes of reoperation are catheter-related complications (migration, coiling, obstruction, breakage, and so forth), which range between 20% and 40%. Intrathecal granuloma formation is a serious complication that has the potential to cause spinal cord compression and neurological devastation. The etiology has not been fully elucidated, but the phenomenon appears to be related to concentration (>25 mg/mL), daily dosage (>10 mg/d), and duration of therapy. However in one review, 39% of morphine-related granulomas were associated with concentrations less than 25 mg/mL, 30% occurred despite doses of under 10 mg/d, and some were noted after within 1 month after initiating therapy [41].

Because of decreased dosing, IT therapy is associated with a lower incidence of many side effects than oral or parenteral use. Nevertheless, the route is not devoid of adverse effects. The most frequent side effects of IT opioids are constipation, urinary retention, nausea/vomiting, sweating, and libido disturbances secondary to hypogonadotrophic hypogonadism [42]. With few exceptions (eg, sweating, peripheral edema, constipation) these adverse effects tend to diminish with time [27]. The mechanism(s) of opioid-induced leg edema is not fully known but may involve partial sympathetic blockade. In one study, Aldrete and da Silva [43] found that among the 22% of FBSS patients who developed lower extremity edema necessitating discontinuation or dose reduction, all had evidence of venous stasis before pump insertion (Table 3).

Local anesthetics

The most widely used spinal analgesics are local anesthetics (LA), which are used to provide both surgical anesthesia and pain relief. The mechanism of action by which LA work is via the blockade of sodium channels, the pivotal event in the depolarization of neurons. As such, LA block the transmission of all neurons, not just the A delta and C fibers responsible for pain.

Numerous studies have documented good intermediate to long-term outcomes mixing LA with opioids and other IT analgesics. Two studies by Sjoberg and colleagues [44,45] conducted in more than 100 cancer patients found the combination of IT morphine and bupivacaine resulted in adequate pain relief in almost 100% of subjects. However, the mean follow-up period in these studies was less than 1 month. In a retrospective study by van Dongen and colleagues [46], the authors found that the addition of IT bupivacaine to opioids resulted in adequate analgesia in 10 of 17 cancer patients who failed IT opioid therapy. The mean follow-up in this study was 112 days. In a later, double-blind, randomized trial comparing IT morphine alone to IT morphine and bupivacaine in 20 cancer patients, the same group found the combination group developed less opioid tolerance than the morphine-only group [47]. The authors concluded the combination of IT bupivacaine and morphine provided synergistic analgesic effects.

Similarly beneficial results have been reported with IT LA-opioid combinations in noncancer pain. Krames [6] reported the addition of bupivacaine to IT opioids either decreased opioid side effects or enhanced analgesia in 77% of 13 patients with nonmalignant pain, with a mean follow-up of

Table 2
Outcomes with intrathecal opioids for noncancer pain

Study	Study type, no. implanted	Follow-up (mean in years)	Relief of pain, n%*	Condition studied	Comments & complications
Plummer et al [23] 1991	Retrospective, 12	0.5	83	Not mentioned	2 pumps explanted for poor pain relief
Krames and Lanning [24] 1993	Retrospective, 16	2.3	81	NO, NP, Mixed (FBSS)	Used MSO4 or hydromorphone; Bupivacaine added in 13/16 patients
Kanoff [25] 1994	Retrospective, 15	0.2–4.0	73	NP, Mixed (FBSS)	2 terminated therapy; 53% excellent relief
Hassenbusch et al [26] 1995	Prospective comparative, 18	0.8–4.7	61	NP	Used MSO4 or sufentanil; 33% re-operation rate; edema resolved in 3 patients after switch to sufentanil
Winkelmuller and winket maller [27] 1996	Retrospective, 120	0.5–6 (mean 3.4)	77	DA, Mixed (FBSS), NP	92% satisfied; 81% improved quality of life
Paice et al [28] 1996	Retrospective physician survey, 296	1.0	95	Mixed (FBSS), NP, NO, DA	Somatic pain improved more than other types; 21.6% mechanical complication rate
Yoshida et al [29] 1996	Retrospective, 18	2.0	25	Mixed (FBSS)	Performed 1.4 additional procedures per patient
Tutak and Doleys [30] 1996	Retrospective, 26	2.0	77	Not mentioned	11 reoperations

Study	Study type, N	Dose	Outcome	Diagnosis	Comments
Angel et al [31] 1998	Prospective observational, 11	0.5–3.0 (mean 2.3)	73	Mixed (FBSS), NP	2 pumps removed for urinary retention
Anderson and Burchiel [32] 1999	Prospective observational, 30	2.0	50% had ≥ 25% pain relief	Mixed (FBSS), NO, DA, NP	20% reoperation rate. Used MSO4 or hydromorphone, with 5 needing bupivacaine
Willis and Odefs [33] 1999	Retrospective study evaluating IT fentanyl after prior opioid failure, 8	2.5	68	Not mentioned	Patients failed IT MSO4 or hydromorphone
Kumar et al [34] 2001	Prospective observational, 16	1–4 (mean 1.5)	NO 57 FBSS 61 DA 75	NO, Mixed (FBSS), DA	3 pumps replaced or explanted; 12 successes
Roberts et al [35] 2001	Retrospective patient survey, 88	3.0	82	Mixed (FBSS), NP, NO	40% of patients required reoperation. 88% satisfaction rate
Anderson et al [36] 2001	Retrospective study evaluating i.t. hydromorphone	0.8	10%; 6 of 16 pts switched to hydromorphone b/c of inadequate analgesia had ≥ 25% pain relief	Mixed (FBSS), NP, NO, DA	All patients failed IT MSO4; Most patients had fewer side effects with hydromorphone
Deer et al [37] 2004	Prospective registry, 136	1.0	62	Mixed (FBSS), NP, NO	21 reoperations to correct mechanical problems; 36 physicians participated
Cherry et al [38] 2003	Case series, 7	2.0–7.0	Angina↓	Angina s/p CABG	Angina improved with IT fentanyl or MSO4

(continued on next page)

Table 2 (continued)

Study	Study type, no. implanted	Follow-up (mean in years)	Relief of pain, n%*	Condition studied	Comments & complications
Thimineur et al [22] 2004	Prospective observational with 2 comparative groups, 31	3	27	Not mentioned	Pain, disability, and depression improved in implanted patients while non-pump recipients worsened
Njee et al [39] 2004	Retrospective, 19	0.3–12.0 mean 4.5	NO 64 FBSS 58 NP 25	Mixed (FBSS), NP, NO	10% infection and catheter dislodgement rate; 90% patient satisfaction
Du Pen et al [40] 2006	Retrospective review of IT hydro-morphone, 24	1.0	25 decrease in VAS	Mixed (FBSS), NO, NP	Average dose increase was 600% in 1 year; only 7 patients had 1-year follow-up data

Abbreviations: CABG, coronary artery bypass surgery; DA, deafferentation pain; FBSS, Failed Back Surgery Syndrome; NO, nociceptive pain; NP, Neuropathic pain; FBSS is listed in parenthesis after "mixed" if the most prevalent cause of mixed neuropathic and nociceptive pain was FBSS.

* Relief of pain = the % of patients with either good or excellent relief or ≥ 50% reduction in pain score.

Table 3
Incidence of side effects with long-term intrathecal opioid therapy, %*

Side effect	%
Constipation	57
Sweating	47
Nausea	42
Urinary retention	37
Vomiting	33
Insomnia/nightmares	28
Impotence	21
Confusion	15
Pruritis	14
Edema	7
Disturbance of libido	6
Fatigue	6
Dry mouth	4
Dizziness	4
Loss of appetite	3
Hypothyroidism	2
Amenorrhea	2
Convulsions	1
Provocation of asthma	1

* *Adapted from* Refs. [27,32,34].

almost 1 year. In a large, retrospective cohort study conducted in 109 patients with FBSS and metastatic cancer of the spine, Deer and colleagues [48] found the combination of opioid and bupivacaine provided superior analgesia and greater patient satisfaction, and was associated with less medication use than IT opioids alone. The average exposure to bupivacaine was 62 weeks. Excellent results were also reported mixing IT bupivacaine with morphine, clonidine, and midazolam in 26 patients with chronic back and/or leg pain [49] (mean follow-up 27 months).

In clinical practice, effective doses of bupivacaine generally range from 3 to 50 mg/d, although there are some reports of daily doses exceeding 100 mg/d [46,50]. Common side effects of IT LA include numbness, paresthesias, weakness, and bowel or bladder dysfunction, all of which can be diminished by using combination therapy.

Calcium channel blockers

Voltage-gated calcium channels play an integral role pain transmission. Numerous classes of voltage-sensitive calcium channels have been identified, which are classified as T, L, N, P, Q, and R subtypes. These channels are characterized by biophysical properties such as sensitivity to pharmacological blocking agents, single-channel conductance kinetics, and voltage-dependence. In animal models of acute pain, there is compelling evidence to support a role for "N-type" calcium channels in nociception, moderate evidence for "L-type" channels, and limited or no evidence for other calcium channels. However, under conditions of persistent nociception induced by chemical, inflammatory, or neuropathic stimuli, all types of calcium channels may play a role in pain maintenance [51,52].

The only calcium channel blocker clinically used to treat chronic pain neuraxially is ziconotide, which blocks N-type calcium channels. Approved by the Food and Drug Administration (FDA) in 2004, ziconotide is a synthetic form of the peptide ω-conotoxin MVIIA isolated from venom produced by the marine snail *Conus magus*. In a multicenter, double-blind, placebo-controlled crossover study evaluating IT ziconotide for the treatment of refractory pain in 111 patients with cancer and AIDS, Staats and colleagues [12] found the treatment group (n = 68) obtained significantly better pain relief than control patients (53.0% versus 17.5%) in all parameters. Thirty-one percent of the ziconotide patients experienced side effects, with the most common being confusion, somnolence, and urinary retention. The observation that there was no loss of efficacy for ziconotide during the 5-day maintenance phase (mean dose 21.8 μg/d) is consistent with animal studies showing a lack of tolerance with calcium channel blockers. In an attempt to reduce side effects, Rauck and colleagues [53] conducted a double-blind, placebo-controlled study using a slower titration schedule and lower maximum dose in 220 patients with chronic, nonmalignant pain (mostly FBSS) refractory to conventional treatment. At the end of the 3-week treatment period, VAS pain scores improved by 15% in the ziconotide group versus 7% in the placebo group. During the treatment period, only 12% of ziconotide patients reported adverse effects.

Although ziconotide is approved only as monotherapy in chronic pain patients who have failed conventional IT therapy, many physicians are using it in combination with opioids and nonopioid analgesics [54]. The major limitations for IT ziconotide are its high cost and the high incidence of side effects, which top 33% in some studies. Adverse effects include psychiatric symptoms, neurological symptoms, cardiovascular events, and gastrointestinal complaints. Currently, IT ziconotide is considered a fourth-line treatment for chronic pain patients [55].

Alpha-2 agonists

Alpha-2 adrenergic receptors play a key role in analgesic effects mediated at peripheral, spinal, and brainstem sites. Several different subtypes of alpha-2 receptors have been identified, although recent studies suggest the alpha-2_A receptor is primarily responsible for analgesia and sedation [56]. Presynaptically, $alpha_2$ agonists bind to receptors on primary afferent neurons, resulting in diminished release of neurotransmitters involved in relaying pain signals. On postsynaptic neurons, they hyperpolarize the cell by increasing potassium conductance through G_i coupled channels. Alpha adrenergic agonists also activate spinal cholinergic neurons, which may potentiate their analgesic effects. In perioperative settings, clonidine has been shown to have synergistic analgesic effects when co-administered with neuraxial LA. However, the evidence that clonidine in combination with opioids is more effective than either agent alone in acute pain settings is weak and inconsistent [57].

The most studied and only FDA-approved alpha-2 agonist for IT use is clonidine. In a prospective, open-label study evaluating combination IT therapy in FBSS, Rainov and colleagues [49] reported good or excellent results at 2-year follow-up in 73% of patients. Sixteen patients received clonidine as part of their IT therapy. Siddall and colleagues [58] conducted a double-blind, placebo-controlled study assessing the efficacy of IT morphine or clonidine, alone or combined, for up to 6 days in 15 patients with central pain secondary to spinal cord injury. The authors found the combination of clonidine and morphine provided significantly better pain relief than saline (37% versus 0% reduction) or either drug alone (20% reduction for morphine, 17% for clonidine). No significant difference was noted in the incidence of side effects.

In addition to prospective studies reporting good outcomes using clonidine in combination with opioids and other analgesics, there are more than 2 dozen reported cases whereby IT clonidine, usually in combination with morphine, provided substantial relief for cancer pain, low back pain (LBP), and even spasticity-related pain in concert with baclofen [59–61]. In 2 retrospective studies, the results are split. Raphael and colleagues [62] reported good outcomes in 74% of patients using combination IT therapy in patients with chronic LBP (clonidine was administered to 27 of 37 patients), with no significant increases in opioid requirements after 2 years of treatment (mean follow-up 4.4 years). However, Ackerman and colleagues [63] reported IT clonidine, with or without opioids, to be of limited value in 15 patients with cancer and chronic nonmalignant pain. The most common side effects of IT clonidine are sedation, hypotension, nausea, and dry mouth. Intrathecal clonidine is recommended in combination with morphine as a second-line therapy for chronic pain [55].

N-methyl-D-aspartate receptor antagonists

Glutamatergic receptors are divided into G-protein coupled (metabotropic) (mGluR) and ion channel (ionotropic) receptors, which include not only N-methyl-D-aspartate (NMDA) receptors, but α-amino-3-hydroxy-5-methylisoxazole-4-propionic acid (AMPA) and kainite receptors. In addition to a binding site for the excitatory neurotransmitter glutamate, the NMDA receptor contains binding sites for the co-agonist glycine, phencyclidine-like compounds, and endogenous protons and polyamines. Following tissue injury, the activation of spinal NMDA receptors induces a state of facilitated processing from repetitive small afferent fiber stimulation, leading to an increased response to high- and low-threshold stimulation, and enhanced receptor field size. This process, known as "wind-up," is responsible for such phenomena such as allodynia and hyperalgesia. In animal studies, selective agonists at the NMDA, AMPA, kainite, and group I mGlu receptors produce spontaneous pain behavior in naïve animals, and allodynia and hyperalgesia in neuropathic and inflammatory models of persistent pain. No AMPA, kainite, or mGluR agonists or antagonists are clinically used in humans.

The most studied NMDA receptor blocker is the noncompetitive antagonist ketamine. In addition to its effects on NMDA receptors, ketamine possesses a plethora of other actions that enhance its analgesic properties. These include blocking non-NMDA glutamate and muscarinic cholinergic receptors, facilitating $GABA_A$ signaling, weakly binding to opioid receptors, and possessing LA and possibly neuroregenerative properties [64].

The results of IT ketamine use in acute and chronic pain have been mixed. In an early study by Bion [65], the administration of hyperbaric ketamine was found to provide adequate anesthesia in 16 patients undergoing lower limb surgery for war injuries. However, more recent studies have reported less-auspicious results. Hawksworth and Serpell [66] found the high incidence of psychomimetic side effects and incomplete anesthesia precluded the use of IT ketamine as a sole anesthetic. Similarly disappointing results were found by Kathirvel and colleagues [67] in 25 women undergoing brachytherapy, and by Togal and colleagues [68] in 40 men undergoing prostate surgery.

For terminal cancer pain, controlled studies and anecdotal experience support the use of IT ketamine in patients refractory to conventional analgesics. Benrath and colleagues [69] reported a patient with metastatic urethral cancer and unremitting neuropathic pain who failed to respond to extremely high doses of IT morphine, bupivacaine, and clonidine. After ketamine was added, a dramatic decrease in pain occurred enabling significant reductions in IT morphine and clonidine, and discontinuation of bupivacaine. Muller and Lemos [70] reported four patients with nociceptive and neuropathic cancer pain who obtained excellent pain relief without tolerance to combination IT therapy with ketamine, morphine, clonidine, and lidocaine. In two of the patients, ketamine was successfully added after tolerance developed to the other three agents. A similar scenario was reported by Vranken and colleagues [71], who described almost complete abolition of neuropathic pain after ketamine was added to the treatment regimen in a cancer patient refractory to IT morphine, bupivacaine, and clonidine. Finally, in a double-blind crossover study comparing the co-administration of low-dose IT ketamine (1 mg) with morphine and IT morphine alone twice daily in 20 patients with terminal cancer, Yang and colleagues [72] found that combination treatment resulted in significantly lower morphine requirements, less rescue medication, and slightly improved pain scores over the 48-hour treatment period. No serious side effects were noted.

The positive reports on the use of IT ketamine for chronic pain remain tempered by questions of neurotoxicity. In the 1990s Karpinski and colleagues [73] reported a terminal cancer patient who received a 3-week IT

infusion of racemic ketamine and was found to have subpial vacuolar myelopathy on autopsy. Stotz and colleagues [74] reported a similar finding 2
years later in another cancer patient following a 7-day trial of IT ketamine.
These reports led subsequent clinicians to limit IT ketamine administration
to preservative-free formulations of the active S(+) enantiomer. However,
Vranken and colleagues [75] recently reported severe histopathological ab-
normalities on postmortem spinal cord examination in a woman with terminal cervical cancer who received excellent pain relief 3 weeks after S(+)
ketamine was added to her IT morphine, bupivacaine, and clonidine regimen. Based on the absence of human toxicology studies, mixed reports of
animal toxicology studies, and anecdotal reports of neurological injury,
IT ketamine should be reserved for terminal patients who fail to derive
pain relief from more conventional analgesics.

Gamma-aminobutyric acid agonists

Three subtypes of the GABA receptor have been identified: $GABA_A$,
$GABA_B$, and $GABA_C$. When these receptors are activated, an influx of
chloride ions enters the cell resulting in hyperpolarization of the cell membrane and decreased neuronal excitability. $GABA_A$ and $GABA_C$ are both
ligand-gated chloride channels, and can be differentiated by location and
response to antagonists. $GABA_A$, the more clinically relevant of the two,
is most prominent in the dorsal horn of the spinal cord.

The $GABA_B$ receptor is a G-protein–linked complex whose activation results in augmentation of potassium channel currents. Like $GABA_A$, GA-
BA_B receptors are found throughout the spinal cord, being located both
pre- and postsynaptically. Presynaptic activation results in decreased neurotransmitter release; postsynaptic activation leads to membrane hyperpolarization and decreased opening of voltage-sensitive calcium channels [76].

Although IT midazolam has been shown to have analgesic efficacy in animal models of visceral, inflammatory somatic, and acute nociception [77],
there are few clinical studies evaluating its use. In a randomized, double-
blind study comparing single-shot epidural steroids with 2 mg of IT midazolam in 25 patients with chronic, mechanical LBP, Serrao and colleagues
[78] reported similar improvement in one half to three quarters of patients
up to 2-months postinjection. However, the use of rescue medication was
less in the midazolam group. Borg and Krijnen [79] treated four patients
with chronic benign neurogenic and musculoskeletal pain refractory to
conventional analgesics with continuous infusions of up to 6 mg/d of IT
midazolam in combination with clonidine or morphine. In all four patients,
long-term combination infusion therapy resulted in nearly complete pain relief. Rainov and colleagues [49] published a pilot study evaluating long-term
treatment outcomes in 26 patients with chronic low back and leg pain
treated with various combinations of IT morphine, bupivacaine, clonidine,
and midazolam (n = 10). Although results were not tabulated by individual

drug combinations, 73% of patients reported good or excellent outcomes. Similar benefits were noted by Yanez and colleagues [80] who reported excellent pain relief in four patients with cancer and noncancer pain poorly responsive to IT morphine. Based on animal and clinical studies, the use of IT midazolam appears to potentiate the analgesic effects of opioids and clonidine.

Animal studies are mixed regarding the toxicity of IT midazolam, with approximately half reporting neurotoxicity [77,81]. Deleterious effects have been demonstrated across a wide range of species and dosages, using mixtures with and without preservatives. However, these reports are balanced by a plethora of similar studies concluding IT midazolam is no more neurotoxic than saline [82,83]. In a randomized study evaluating the effects of adding 2 mg of midazolam to LA in 1100 patients undergoing spinal anesthesia, Tucker and colleagues [84] found no increase in postoperative neurological symptoms in patients who received combination treatment. The most common side effect of IT midazolam is dose-dependent sedation, with motor weakness occurring only at high doses. Midazolam is currently a fourth-line IT treatment for chronic pain [55].

Preclinical studies with $GABA_B$ agonists in animal models of acute and persistent nociception found that $GABA_B$ agonists such as baclofen produce antinociception and anti-allodynia at doses that do not impair motor function [85]. In a recent review, Slonimski and colleagues [86] eloquently detailed the preclinical evidence demonstrating efficacy for IT baclofen in spasm-induced, neuropathic, sympathetically maintained and acute pain. Intrathecal baclofen has been used to treat spasticity since the mid-1980s, and is FDA-approved for this indication. In a Cochrane review of pharmacological interventions for spinal cord injury (SCI)-induced spasticity, Tarrico and colleagues [87] concluded only IT baclofen has been proven effective. In a similar meta-analysis conducted for spasticity associated with multiple sclerosis (MS), Beard and colleagues [88] found good evidence to support only IT baclofen and botulinum toxin. These findings are consistent with reviews evaluating treatments for spasticity derived from other etiologies.

Clinical studies have also demonstrated IT baclofen to be effective for a wide array of other pain conditions. In a randomized, double-blind cross-over trial, seven women with complex regional pain syndrome (CRPS) were given bolus injections of either baclofen 25, 50, or 75 μg or saline [89]. No difference was found between 25 μg and saline injections. With higher doses, six of seven patients had complete or partial resolution of symptoms and proceeded to pump implantation. Three months postimplant, three women had regained normal hand function and two the ability to walk. Three had marked reductions in pain, four in paresthesias and two in numbness. The beneficial effects of IT baclofen in CRPS is supported by the work of Zuniga and colleagues [90], who reported two cases of refractory CRPS type I successfully treated with baclofen. In both patients, dramatic improvements in autonomic symptoms, and spontaneous and evoked pain were noted.

Intrathecal baclofen is considered the gold standard for spasticity, but anecdotal evidence suggests it may alleviate central pain as well. In a double-blind, placebo-controlled study by Herman and colleagues [91] conducted in patients with MS and SCI, the authors found significant reductions in dysesthetic and spasm-related pain, but no effect on evoked pain. These results are supported by Taira and colleagues [92] who found 9 of 14 patients with central pain secondary to stroke or SCI experienced significant reductions in spontaneous pain, allodynia, and hyperalgesia following an IT baclofen bolus. They are in contrast to the findings of Loubser and Akman, [93] who found that while musculoskeletal pain decreased in a large majority of SCI patients 1 year after initiation of IT baclofen, only 22% experienced a significant decline in neurogenic pain.

In addition to chronic pain associated with spasticity, IT baclofen has been reported to relieve neuropathic pain secondary to FBSS, amputation, and plexopathy [94]. In a recent case series conducted in patients with refractory neuropathic pain, Lind and colleagues [95] treated seven patients with IT baclofen pumps and spinal cord stimulation and four with baclofen alone. Although both groups obtained significant pain relief, a greater reduction in pain scores occurred in the combination group (mean follow-up 35 months).

The most common side effects associated with IT baclofen are drowsiness, cognitive impairment, weakness, gastrointestinal complaints, and sexual dysfunction [96]. Baclofen is currently considered a fourth-line treatment for chronic pain [55] (Table 4).

Table 4
Dose range and evidence for efficacy and commonly used intrathecal analgesic agents

Drug	Typical dose range	Clinical evidence for efficacy
Morphine	1–20 mg/d	Strong evidence for cancer pain. Moderate evidence for nonmalignant pain.
Hydromorphone	0.5–10 mg/d	Same as morphine.
Fentanyl	0.02–0.3 mg/d	Same as morphine.
Bupivacaine	4–30 mg/d	Strong evidence for cancer pain. Moderate evidence for nonmalignant pain.
Midazolam	0.2–6 mg/d	Weak evidence for chronic back pain. Anecdotal evidence for neuropathic pain.
Clonidine	0.03–1 mg/d	Weak evidence for cancer pain. Moderate evidence for back pain. Weak evidence for central pain. Moderate evidence for neuropathic pain.
Ketamine	1–50 mg/d	Moderate evidence for cancer pain. Weak evidence for neuropathic pain.
Baclofen	0.05–0.8 mg/d	Strong evidence for muscle spasm–related pain. Weak evidence for central pain. Moderate evidence for neuropathic pain.

Summary

Since the advent of implantable IT drug delivery systems over 25 years ago, numerous advances have been made with regard to system technology, pharmacology, and patient selection. Whereas strong evidence exists for the use of IT therapy for cancer pain, the evidence supporting long-term efficacy in noncancer pain is less convincing. However, in carefully selected patients, combination therapy appears to provide the ideal balance between efficacy and side effects, at least for intermediate-term outcomes. Areas most ripe for future investigation include which pain conditions are most amenable to IT therapy, the long-term efficacy of infusion therapy for noncancer pain, particularly in regard to functional improvement, delineating which drug combinations provide the best balance between efficacy and adverse effects, and conducting preclinical and clinical safety studies on promising analgesics such as ketamine and midazolam.

References

[1] Pert CB, Snyder S. Opiate receptor: demonstration in nervous tissue. Science 1973;179(77): 1011–4.

[2] Terenius L. Characteristics of the "receptor" for narcotic analgesics in synaptic plasma membrane fractions from rat brain. Acta Pharmacol Toxicol (Copenh) 1973;33(5):377–84.

[3] Yaksh TL, Rudy TA. Studies on the direct spinal action of narcotics in the production of analgesia in the rat. J Pharmacol Exp Ther 1977;202(2):411–28.

[4] Wang JK, Nauss LA, Thomas JE. Pain relief by intrathecally applied morphine in man. Anesthesiology 1979;50(2):149–51.

[5] Foley KM. Treatment of cancer pain. N Engl J Med 1985;313(2):84–95.

[6] Krames ES. Intrathecal infusional therapies for intractable pain: patient management guidelines. J Pain Symptom Manage 1993;8(1):36–46.

[7] Kalso E, Edwards JE, Moore RA, et al. Opioids in chronic non-cancer pain: systematic review of efficacy and safety. Pain 2004;112(3):372–80.

[8] Ives TJ, Chelminski PR, Hammett-Stabler CA, et al. Predictors of opioid misuse in patients with chronic pain: a prospective cohort study. BMC Health Serv Res 2006;6:46.

[9] Ballantyne JC, Mao J. Opioid therapy for chronic pain. N Engl J Med 2003;349(20): 1943–53.

[10] Webster LR, Webster RM. Predicting aberrant behaviors in opioid-treated patients: preliminary validation of the Opioid Risk Tool. Pain Med 2006;6(6):432–42.

[11] Kittelberger KP, Buchheit TE, Rice SF. Self-extraction of intrathecal pump opioid. Anesthesiology 2004;101(3):807.

[12] Staats PS, Yearwood T, Charapata SG, et al. Intrathecal ziconotide in the treatment of refractory pain in patients with cancer or AIDS: a randomized controlled trial. JAMA 2004; 291(1):63–70.

[13] Akil H, Watson SJ, Young E, et al. Endogenous opioids: biology and function. Annu Rev Neurosci 1984;7:223–55.

[14] Reisine T. Opiate receptors. Neuropharmacology 1995;34(5):463–72.

[15] Ocana M, Cendan CM, Cobos EJ, et al. Potassium channels and pain: present realities and future opportunities. Eur J Pharmacol 2004;500(1–3):203–19.

[16] Smith TJ, Staats PS, Deer T, et al. Implantable Drug Delivery Systems Study Group. Randomized clinical trial of an implantable drug delivery system compared with comprehensive

medical management for refractory cancer pain. Impact on pain, drug-related toxicity, and survival. J Clin Oncol 2002;20(19):4040–9.

[17] Rauck RL, Cherry D, Boyer MF, et al. Long-term intrathecal opioid therapy with a patient-activated, implanted delivery system for the treatment of refractory cancer pain. J Pain 2003; 4(8):441–7.

[18] Zeppetella G, O'Doherty CA, Collins S. Prevalence and characteristics of breakthrough pain in patients with non-malignant terminal disease admitted to a hospice. Palliat Med 2001; 15(3):243–6.

[19] Portenoy RK, Hagen NA. Breakthrough pain: definition, prevalence and characteristics. Pain 1990;41(3):273–81.

[20] Idanpaan-Heikkila JJ, Guilbaud G. Pharmacological studies on a rat model of trigeminal neuropathic pain: baclofen, but not carbamazepine, morphine or tricyclic antidepressants, attenuates the allodynia-like behavior. Pain 1999;79(2–3):281–90.

[21] Hanks GW, Forbes K. Opioid responsiveness. Acta Anaesthesiol Scand 1997;41(1 Pt 2): 154–8.

[22] Thimineur MA, Kravitz E, Vodapally MS. Intrathecal opioid treatment for chronic non-malignant pain: a 3-year prospective study. Pain 2004;109(3):242–9.

[23] Plummer JL, Cherry DA, Cousins MJ, et al. Long-term spinal administration of morphine in cancer and non-cancer pain: a retrospective study. Pain 1991;44(3):215–20.

[24] Krames ES, Lanning RM. Intrathecal infusional analgesia for nonmalignant pain: analgesic efficacy of intrathecal opioid with or without bupivacaine. J Pain Symptom Manage 1993; 8(8):539–48.

[25] Kanoff RB. Intraspinal delivery of opiates by an implantable, programmable pump in patients with chronic, intractable pain of nonmalignant origin. J Am Osteopath Assoc 1994; 94(6):487–93.

[26] Hassenbusch SJ, Stanton-Hicks M, Covington EC, et al. Long-term intraspinal infusions of opiods in the treatment of neuropathic pain. J Pain Symptom Manage 1995;10(7): 527–43.

[27] Winkelmuller M, Winkelmuller W. Long-term effects of continuous intrathecal opioid treatment in chronic pain of nonmalignant etiology. J Neurosurg 1996;85(3):458–67.

[28] Paice JA, Penn RD, Shott S. Intraspinal morphine for chronic pain: a retrospective, multi-center study. J Pain Symptom Manage 1996;11(2):71–80.

[29] Yoshida GM, Nelson RW, Capen DA. Evaluation of contiuous intraspinal narcotic analgesia for chronic pain from benign causes. Am J Orthop 1996;25(10):693–4.

[30] Tutak U, Doleys DM. Intrathecal infusion systems for treatment of chronic low back and leg pain of noncancer origin. South Med J 1996;89(3):295–300.

[31] Angel IF, Gould HJ Jr, Carey ME. Intrathecal morphine pump as a treatment option in chronic pain of nonmalignant origin. Surg Neurol 1998;49(1):92–9.

[32] Anderson VC, Burchiel KJ. A prospective study of long-term intrathecal morphine in the management of chronic nonmalignant pain. Neurosurgery 1999;44(2):289–300.

[33] Willis KD, Doleys DM. The effects of long-term intraspinal infusion therapy with noncancer pain patients: evaluation of patient, significant-other, and clinic staff appraisals. Neuromodulation 1999;2(4):241–53.

[34] Kumar K, Kelly M, Pirlot T. Continuous intrathecal morphine treatment for chronic pain of nonmalignant etiology: long-term benefits and efficacy. Surg Neurol 2001;55: 79–88.

[35] Roberts LJ, Finch PM, Goucke CR, et al. Outcome of intrathecal opioids in chronic non-cancer pain. Eur J Pain 2001;5(4):353–61.

[36] Anderson VC, Cooke B, Burchiel KJ. Intrathecal hydromorphone for chronic nonmalignant pain: a retrospective study. Pain Med 2001;2(4):287–97.

[37] Deer T, Chapple I, Classen A, et al. Intrathecal drug delivery for treatment of chronic low back pain: report from the National Outcomes Registry for low back pain. Pain Med 2004;5(1):6–13.

[38] Cherry DA, Gourlay GK, Eldredge KA. Management of chronic intractable angina: spinal opioids offer an alternative therapy. Pain 2003;102(1–2):163–6.
[39] Njee TB, Irthum B, Roussel P, et al. Intrathecal morphine infusion for chronic non-malignant pain: a multiple center retrospective study. Neuromodulation 2004;7(4): 249–59.
[40] Du Pen S, Du Pen A, Hillyer J. Intrathecal hydromorphone for intractable nonmalignant pain: a retrospective study. Pain Med 2006;7(1):10–5.
[41] Yaksh TL, Hassenbusch S, Burchiel K, et al. Inflammatory masses associated with intrathe-cal drug infusion: a review of preclinical evidence and human data. Pain Med 2002;3(4): 300–12.
[42] Paice JA, Penn RD, Ryan W. Altered sexual function and decreased testosterone in patients receiving intraspinal opioids. J Pain Symtom Manage 1994;9(2):126–31.
[43] Aldrete JA, Couto da Silva JM. Leg edema from intrathecal opiate infusions. Eur J Pain 2000;4(4):361–5.
[44] Sjoberg M, Nitescu P, Appelgren L, et al. Long-term intrathecal morphine and bupivacaine in patients with refractory cancer pain. Results from a morphine:bupivacaine dose regimen of 0.5:4.75 mg/ml. Anesthesiology 1994;80(2):284–97.
[45] Sjoberg M, Appelgren L, Einarsson S, et al. Long-term intrathecal morphine and bupiva-caine in "refractory" cancer pain. I. Results from the first series of 52 patients. Acta Anaes-thesiol Scand 1991;35(1):30–43.
[46] van Dongen RT, Crul BJ, De Bock M. Long-term intrathecal infusion of morphine and mor-phine/bupivacaine mixtures in the treatment of cancer pain: a retrospective analysis of 51 cases. Pain 1993;55(1):119–23.
[47] van Dongen RT, Crul BJ, van Egmond J. Intrathecal coadministration of bupivacaine diminishes morphine dose progression during long-term intrathecal infusion in cancer patients. Clin J Pain 1999;15(3):166–72.
[48] Deer TR, Caraway DL, Kim CK, et al. Clinical experience with intrathecal bupivacaine in combination with opioid for the treatment of chronic pain related to failed back surgery syndrome and metastatic cancer pain of the spine. Spine J 2002;2(4):274–8.
[49] Rainov NG, Heidecke V, Burkert W. Long-term intrathecal infusion of drug combinations for chronic back and leg pain. J Pain Symptom Manage 2001;22(4):862–71.
[50] Berde CB, Sethna NF, Conrad LS. Subarachnoid bupivacaine analgesia for seven months for a patient with a spinal cord tumor. Anesthesiology 1990;72(6):1094–6.
[51] Vanegas H, Schaible H. Effects of antagonists to high-threshold calcium channels upon spinal mechanisms of pain, hyperalgesia and allodynia. Pain 2000;85(1–2):9–18.
[52] McGivern JG. Targeting N-type and T-type calcium channels for the treatment of pain. Drug Discov Today 2006;11(5–6):245–53.
[53] Rauck RL, Wallace MS, Leong MS, et al. A randomized, double-blind, placebo-controlled study of intrathecal ziconotide in adults with severe chronic pain. J Pain Symptom Manage 2006;31(5):393–406.
[54] Thompson JC, Dunbar E, Laye RR. Treatment challenges and complications with zicono-tide monotherapy in established pump patients. Pain Physician 2006;9(2):147–52.
[55] Hassenbusch SJ, Portenoy RK, Cousins M, et al. Polyanalgesic Consensus Conference 2003: an update on the management of pain by intraspinal drug delivery—report of an expert panel. J Pain Symptom Manage 2004;27(6):540–63.
[56] Kamibayashi T, Maze M. Clinical uses of alpha 2-adrenergic agonists. Anesthesiology 2000; 93(5):1345–9.
[57] Walker SM, Goudas LC, Cousins MJ, et al. Combination spinal analgesic chemotherapy: a systematic review. Anesth Analg 2002;95(3):674–715.
[58] Siddall PJ, Molloy AR, Walker S, et al. The efficacy of intrathecal morphine and clonidine in the treatment of pain after spinal cord injury. Anesth Analg 2000;91(6):1493–8.
[59] Uhle EI, Becker R, Gatscher S, et al. Continuous intrathecal clonidine administration for the treatment of neuropathic pain. Stereotact Funct Neurosurg 2000;75(4):167–75.

[60] Eisenach JC, De Kock M, Klimscha W. Alpha (2)-adrenergic agonists for regional anesthesia. A clinical review of clonidine (1984–1995). Anesthesiology 1996;85(3):655–74.

[61] Middleton JW, Siddall PJ, Walker S. Intrathecal clonidine and baclofen in the management of spasticity and neuropathic pain following spinal cord injury: a case study. Arch Phys Med Rehabil 1996;77(8):824–6.

[62] Raphael JH, Southall JL, Gnanadurai TV, et al. Long-term experience with implanted intrathecal drug administration systems for failed back syndrome and chronic mechanical low back pain. BMC Musculoskelet Disord 2002;3:17.

[63] Ackerman LL, Follett KA, Rosenquist RW. Long-term outcomes during treatment of chronic pain with intrathecal clonidine or clonidine/opioid combinations. J Pain Symptom Manage 2003;26(1):668–77.

[64] Cohen SP, Chang AS, Larkin T, et al. The IV ketamine test: a predictive response tool for an oral dextromethorphan treatment regimen in neuropathic pain. Anesth Analg 2004;99(6): 1753–9.

[65] Bion JF. Intrathecal ketamine for war surgery. A preliminary study under field conditions. Anaesthesia 1984;39(10):1023–8.

[66] Hawksworth C, Serpell M. Intrathecal anesthesia with ketamine. Reg Anesth Pain Med 1998;23(3):283–8.

[67] Kathirvel S, Sadhasivam S, Saxena A, et al. Effects of intrathecal ketamine added to bupivacaine for spinal anaesthesia. Anaesthesia 2000;55(9):899–904.

[68] Togal T, Demirbilek S, Koroglu A, et al. Effects of S(+) ketamine added to bupivacaine for spinal anaesthesa for prostate surgery in elderly patients. Eur J Anaesthesiol 2004;21(3): 193–7.

[69] Benrath J, Scharbert G, Gustorff B, et al. Long-term intrathecal S(+)-ketamine in a patient with cancer-related neuropathic pain. Br J Anaesth 2005;95(2):247–9.

[70] Muller A, Lemos D. Cancer pain: beneficial effect of ketamine addition to spinal administration of morphine-clonidine-lidocaine mixture. Ann Fr Anesth Reanim 1996;15(3):271–6.

[71] Vranken JH, van der Vegt MH, Kal JE, et al. Treatment of neuropathic cancer pain with continuous intrathecal administration of S + -ketamine. Acta Anaesthesiol Scand 2004; 48(2):249–52.

[72] Yang CY, Wong CS, Chang JY, et al. Intrathecal ketamine reduces morphine requirements in patients with terminal cancer pain. Can J Anaesth 1996;43(4):379–83.

[73] Karpinski N, Dunn J, Hansen L, et al. Subpial vacuolar myelopathy after intrathecal ketamine: report of a case. Pain 1997;73(1):103–5.

[74] Stotz M, Oehen HP, Gerber H. Histological findings after long-term infusion of intrathecal ketamine for chronic pain: a case report. J Pain Symptom Manage 1999;18(3):223–8.

[75] Vranken JH, Troost D, Wegener JT, et al. Neuropathological findings after continuous intrathecal administration of S(+)-ketamine for the management of neuropathic cancer pain. Pain 2005;117(1–2):231–5.

[76] Bowery NG. GABA$_B$ receptor pharmacology. Annu Rev Pharmacol Toxicol 1993;33: 109–47.

[77] Yaksh TL, Allen JW. The use of intrathecal midazolam in humans: A case study of process. Anesth Analg 2004;98(6):1536–45.

[78] Serrao JM, Marks RL, Morley SJ, et al. Intrathecal midazolam for the treatment of chronic mechanical low back pain; a controlled comparison with epidural steroid in a pilot study. Pain 1992;48(1):5–12.

[79] Borg PA, Krijnen JH. Long-term intrathecal administration of midazolam and clonidine. Clin J Pain 1996;12(1):63–8.

[80] Yanez A, Peleteiro R, Camba MA. [Intrathecal administration of morphine, midazolam, and their combination in 4 patients with chronic pain.] Rev Esp Anestesiol Reanim 1992; 39(1):40–2 [in Spanish].

[81] Ugur B, Basaloglu K, Yurtseven T, et al. Neurotoxicity with single dose intrathecal midazolam administration. Eur J Anaesthesiol 2005;22(12):907–12.

[82] Bahar M, Cohen ML, Grinshpon Y, et al. Spinal anaesthesia with midazolam in the rat. Can J Anaesth 1997;44(2):208–15.

[83] Johansen MJ, Gradert TL, Satterfield WC. Safety of continuous intrathecal midazolam infusion in the sheep model. Anesth Analg 2004;98(6):1528–35.

[84] Tucker AP, Lai C, Nadeson R, et al. Intrathecal midazolam. I. A cohort study investigating safety. Anesth Analg 2004;98(6):1512–20.

[85] Hwang JH, Yaksh TL. The effect of spinal GABA receptor agonists on tactile allodynia in a surgically-induced neuropathic pain model in the rat. Pain 1997;70(1):15–22.

[86] Slonimski M, Abram S, Zuniga R. Intrathecal baclofen in pain management. Reg Anesth Pain Med 2004;29(3):269–76.

[87] Taricco M, Adone R, Pagliacci C, et al. Pharmacological interventions for spasticity following spinal cord injury. Cochrane Database Syst Rev 2000;2:CD00131.

[88] Beard S, Hunn A, Wight J. Treatments for spasticity and pain in multiple sclerosis: a systematic review. Health Technol Assess 2003;7(40):1–111.

[89] van Hilten BJ, van de Beek WT, Hoff JI, et al. Intrathecal baclofen for the treatment of dystonia in patients with reflex sympathetic dystrophy. N Engl J Med 2000;343(9):625–30.

[90] Zuniga RE, Perera S, Abram SE. Intrathecal baclofen: a useful agent in the treatment of well-established complex regional pain syndrome. Reg Anesth Pain Med 2002;27(1):90–3.

[91] Herman RM, D'Luzansky JC, Ippolito R. Intrathecal baclofen suppresses central pain in patients with spinal lesions. Clin J Pain 1992;8(4):338–45.

[92] Taira T, Kawamura H, Tanikawa T, et al. A new approach to control central deafferentation pain: spinal intrathecal baclofen. Stereotactic Funct Neurosurg 1995;65(1–4):101–5.

[93] Loubser PG, Akman NM. Effects of intrathecal baclofen on chronic spinal cord injury pain. J Pain Symptom Manage 1996;12(4):241–7.

[94] Zuniga RE, Schlicht CR, Abram SE. Intrathecal baclofen is analgesic in patients with chronic pain. Anesthesiology 2000;92(3):876–80.

[95] Lind G, Meyerson BA, Winter J, et al. Intrathecal baclofen as adjuvant therapy to enhance the effect of spinal cord stimulation in neuropathic pain: a pilot study. Eur J Pain 2004;8(4):377–83.

[96] Denys P, Mane M, Azouvi P. Side effects of chronic intrathecal baclofen on erection and ejaculation in patients with spinal cord lesions. Arch Phys Med Rehabil 1998;79(5):494–6.

ELSEVIER
SAUNDERS

THE MEDICAL
CLINICS
OF NORTH AMERICA

Med Clin N Am 91 (2007) 271–286

Interventional Approaches
to Pain Management

John D. Markman, MD[a,b,*], Annie Philip, MD[a]

[a]Department of Anesthesiology, University of Rochester School of Medicine and Dentistry,
601 Elmwood Avenue, Rochester, NY 14642, USA
[b]The Pain Management Center at University of Rochester Medical Center,
Rochester, NY 14642, USA

Interventional approaches remain a mainstay of chronic pain treatment despite the many challenges to the study of their efficacy. When less invasive analgesic modalities provide inadequate relief, these techniques often play a complementary role. Interventional strategies typically target the neural structures that are presumed to mediate the experience of pain. The varied mechanisms of action range from reversible blockade with local anesthetics, to augmentation with spinal cord stimulation, and ablation with radiofrequency energy or neurolytic agents. Other techniques access intraspinal routes of medication delivery to improve an effective drug's therapeutic index. Many of the most common approaches are uniquely suited to offer rapid, potent, local control of pain with reduced systemic side effects.

Clinical indications for interventional pain management strategies encompass a broad range of conditions, from intractable neuropathic symptoms caused by advanced cancer to chronic, noncancer pain involving the spine. Each technique bears specific risks that pertain to its anatomic targets and therapeutic mechanism of action. Review of the evidence for the interventions considered raises practical issues common to virtually all procedures for chronic pain: (1) the validity of extending an indication for cancer pain to noncancer pain, (2) the timing and repeated use of a strategy with temporary benefit in the perioperative setting to a chronic pain condition, (3) the impact of neuroplasticity on the development of tolerance to analgesic effect, and (4) the clinical significance of a reduction in pain intensity in the absence of demonstrable function or benefit. This article traces

    * Corresponding author. Department of Anesthesiology, University of Rochester School of Medicine and Dentistry, 601 Elmwood Avenue, Box 604, Rochester, NY 14642.
    E-mail address: john_markman@urmc.rochester.edu (J.D. Markman).

0025-7125/07/$ - see front matter © 2007 Elsevier Inc. All rights reserved.
doi:10.1016/j.mcna.2006.10.015
medical.theclinics.com

the rationale and pivotal evidence for some representative, common interventional procedures, with the aim of helping nonspecialist physicians identify the patients most likely to benefit from these approaches.

Historical context and general considerations

The discovery of the local anesthetic properties of cocaine and the characterization of methods for subcutaneous and spinal injection in the late nineteenth century laid the groundwork for today's interventional pain management strategies [1]. These techniques were refined in the early twentieth century and were increasingly deployed beyond the operating room by the end of World War II. Anesthesiology-based "nerve block" clinics of that era have given way to an integrated treatment approach to chronic pain that incorporates psychologic and rehabilitative techniques [2].

A revolution in synthetic chemistry has paralleled refinements in neural blockade. The result has been a growing armamentarium of systemic analgesics, including acetaminophen, nonsteroidal anti-inflammatory drugs, semisynthetic and synthetic opioid analgesics, and the heterogenous group of medications known as adjuvants. Many of the medications in this latter group were developed for conditions such as epilepsy, and only later were found to have analgesic properties in conditions such as neuropathic pain [3]. In a similar way, interventional techniques shown to have temporary benefit in the perioperative setting have been extrapolated to chronic pain treatment. Despite the emergence of myriad pharmacologic and nonpharmacologic methods to treat chronic pain in an interdisciplinary environment, many of these are not well-tolerated or do not alleviate symptoms sufficiently [4]. The potential benefit of local and neuraxial approaches is often greatest when pain remains poorly controlled with pharmacologic and nonpharmacologic strategies.

Few placebo-controlled studies of invasive approaches for the treatment of chronic pain have been carried out. Factors complicating the study of procedures include the absence of consensus standards for block technique; the ethical questions and patient enrollment challenges posed by placebo-controlled research; limitations to treatment blinding; and the difficulty of quantifying psychosocial variables, such as litigation and family support, that influence treatment outcome [5]. As a consequence, the procedures developed for pain management have not been subject to placebo-controlled evaluation approaching the scale of newer pharmacologic agents. This limitation is balanced by the fact that most interventional techniques and associated drugs have been adapted from the perioperative context where their use is commonplace and the risks are well-characterized [6].

Symptom- and disease-based paradigms, rather than a mechanism-based understanding of pain, commonly inform treatment decisions. Drugs such as a gabapentin, for which there is strong evidence of analgesic benefit in a few neuropathic conditions, are used frequently to treat related symptom patterns [7]. Extrapolation of clinical trial data and individualized assessment of treatment response appears to be the norm in pharmacologic and procedural decision making alike [8]. For example, spinal cord stimulation is used to treat intractable lower extremity chronic pain characterized as "burning" following laminectomy and for a similar symptom characterization in complex regional pain syndrome [9,10]. Evidence does not show that these symptom patterns share a common underlying mechanism, despite the similar features. Patients undergo a defined trial of neuroaugmentation with different configurations of stimulation, just as they might engage in a titrated trial of a medication such as gabapentin. Treatment response, however defined, is not tantamount to a precise disclosure of the underlying pathophysiology of pain.

The diagnostic role of neural blockade is often overshadowed by its potential therapeutic benefit. The reversible interruption of neural conduction with local anesthetic may be used to disclose the localization and relative contribution of different structures along the nociceptive pathways that mediate the experience of pain. To some extent, this role has increased in importance because the widespread use of detailed imaging studies such as MRI and CT are sensitive and specific for anatomic changes but not for the presence of pain [11]. This problem is magnified when imaging correlation with patient report of symptoms is poor. Neural blockade may help determine a peripheral source of pain from a neuroma or entrapped nerve not amenable to visualization with advanced techniques. Blockade may assist in differentiating a local site of pain from a knee joint from that referred in a dermatomal distribution due to lumbar root injury. Alternatively, regional anesthetic techniques may distinguish somatic from visceral pain, as in certain pelvic pain syndromes. The diagnostic value of local anesthetic blockade for localization of chronic pain of spinal origin has limitations. For example, attempts to enrich study cohorts for the treatment of facet syndrome with diagnostic blocks have been hampered by low sensitivity and specificity [12]. Repetition of diagnostic blocks and the controversial use of sham blocks in the setting of clinical trials have been shown to improve sensitivity and specificity [13].

Intraspinal opioid delivery

Since the 1970s, when endogenous opioids and opioid receptors in the dorsal horn of the spinal cord were first identified, attempts have been made to optimize this form of therapy by delivering opioids centrally. In the small minority of cancer patients for whom oral and systemic opioid medication does not provide adequate pain control despite opioid rotation, changing the route of administration may enhance efficacy and minimize systemic side effects [14,15]. The principal benefit of intraspinal delivery appears to be the reduction in opioid side effects, rather than improved analgesia [16]. Adoption of these approaches has grown over the past 2 decades;

as many as 20% of patients who had cancer were treated with spinal opioids in one series [17]. In patients who have cancer, the timing of intervention has proved to be among the most difficult clinical questions. Intolerance to systemic opioids, poorly controlled incident pain with movement, and intractable pain caused by neuroinvasive lesions, such as involvement of a plexus, are among the most common indications. The evidence for the use of these approaches in cancer pain is far more robust than for chronic noncancer pain where the risk-benefit balance may become less favorable with the course of time.

The delivery systems that introduce medication into the epidural and intrathecal spaces are varied. These include programmable, implanted pumps; implanted accessible reservoir systems; and tunneled, exteriorized catheters [18]. Epidural and external pump strategies have the greatest value when life expectancy is short (ie, <2 months). The type of trial that should precede implantation of a permanent device remains an unsettled issue and considerable variation in practice persists. In addition to morphine, which was until recently the only Food and Drug Administration–approved agent, dilute local anesthetic preparations and clonidine have been used effectively to augment analgesia [19]. The synergistic effects may confer greater relief in patients who have poorly controlled, incident pain and neuropathic pain [20]. Recently, intrathecal ziconotide, a selective N-type voltage-sensitive Ca^{2+} channel blocking agent, has demonstrated a significant reduction in pain in patients who have cancer or AIDS [21]. Intraspinal delivery systems enable logarithmic scale reductions in medication dosing, but require close monitoring of patients, especially early in the titration phases. The care of patients with tunneled subcutaneous catheters involves routine prophylactic measures (eg, bacterial filters, exit-site care) and monitoring for infection.

The preponderance of evidence supporting intraspinal opioid delivery is based on nonrandomized, uncontrolled series [22]. Two large studies have demonstrated improved analgesic efficacy and reduced toxic side effects in patients requiring a high dose of oral morphine [23,24]. The largest, randomized, prospective clinical trial compared an implantable drug delivery system with comprehensive medical management for refractory cancer pain (eg, Visual Analogue Scale [VAS] pain score ≥5 on a 0–10 scale). Clinical success was defined as a greater than or equal to 20% reduction in VAS scores, or equivalent analgesia with a greater than or equal to 20% reduction in opioid toxicity. Sixty of the seventy-one patients (84.5%) in the intraspinal treatment group achieved clinical success, compared with fifty-one of seventy-two comprehensive medical management patients. Patients receiving intrathecal therapy reported a significant reduction in fatigue and a depressed level of consciousness. Limitations of this study included the absence of controls for radiotherapy and chemotherapy, the younger age of the participants relative to the typical cancer population, and an inconsistent comparative benefit of the intrathecal route of delivery at different time points during the trial. Tight adherence to the algorithm for comprehensive medical management in the setting of a clinical trial produced a marked improvement in pain control. In a separate small, brief, double-blinded, crossover study of epidural and subcutaneous morphine, there was an advantage with regard to analgesia and a reduction in dose and side effects compared with oral morphine [25].

Lack of validated criteria for selection of patients and long-term data to evaluate the efficacy of intrathecal drug delivery systems in chronic, non-cancer pain have limited adoption of this technology. Patients who have multiple types of intractable pain with nociceptive and neuropathic mechanisms inferred are described as the candidates most likely to benefit, but investigators who report treatment success in most cases concede patient selection remains difficult. A series by Kumar [26] reported significant opioid dose escalation with reduced analgesic benefit at 2 years. Favorable retrospective evidence from 12-month follow-up was seen in a small series of patients receiving intrathecal hydromorphone [27]. In one intriguing study, pump recipients demonstrated improvements in pain, mood, and function from baseline to 3 years following implant [28]. Despite this apparent benefit, these patients experienced a decline in function, an increase in self-rated pain, and more mood disturbances, compared with new patients referred to a pain specialist's practice. This finding suggests that pain severity remains high in these patients, despite the intervention. Uncontrolled studies with open follow-up have suggested benefit from long-term intrathecal treatment of spasticity and spasm-related pain with baclofen, a γ-aminobutyric acid agonist [29].

The risks and costs of intraspinal opioids exceed that of systemic opioids. The most common catheter-related problems, occurring in up to 25% of patients, include: kinking, obstruction, disconnection, and granuloma formation at the catheter tip with prolonged, high-rate infusion. Retrospective studies have shown the incidence of delayed respiratory depression with intrathecal narcotics to be 4% to 7% and with epidural infusion to be 0.25% to 0.5%. Pruritus occurs in up to 20% of patients, and urinary retention in as high as 15%. In one series of epidural delivery where nearly three quarters of patients achieved satisfactory relief, the investigators cautioned that the benefit was offset by the rate of deep infection, including epidural abscess, which reached 13% of patients [30].

Neurolytic blockade

Celiac plexus neurolysis in intra-abdominal cancer

Pancreatic adenocarcinoma and cancer of the upper abdominal viscera are commonly associated with severe, poorly controlled pain [31]. In pancreatic cancer, the pain is present early in the course of the disease and the prognosis is poor. Upper abdomen pain is mediated by the afferent nociceptive fibers that travel with the sympathetic fibers of the splanchnic nerves arising from T5-T12 and the parasympathetic efferent fibers that together form the celiac plexus. The ganglia are situated in the retroperitoneal space adjacent to the L1 vertebral body. Since the initial description almost a century ago, focal destruction of this nerve tissue has undergone numerous refinements that have improved both safety and efficacy [32]. The approach is reserved for pain associated with life-limiting illness largely because durable benefit in noncancer abdominal pain has not been demonstrated convincingly [33]. As with other interventional approaches in cancer pain management, some experts advocate the early use of these techniques because of superior pain relief, reduction in opioid side effects, and even improvement in quality-of-life measures [34]. The evidence is strongest for comparable relief with a reduction in opioid side effects.

Neurolytic celiac plexus blockade is the most extensively studied ablative procedure for the treatment of cancer pain. The most commonly used agent is alcohol, 50% to 100%, which provokes an extraction of lipids and a precipitation of proteins [35]. Phenol is also used for neurolysis and may carry a reduced risk of postinjection neuritis, but higher viscosity makes it more challenging to inject. With either agent, the variable duration of analgesia is typically on the order of months. The block has been performed using surface landmarks, fluoroscopy, CT, and ultrasound guidance. Numerous variations on the percutaneous, bilateral, retrocrural approach have been introduced over the past 2 decades, including transcrural, single-needle transaortic, and anterior, transabdominal approaches [36]. Most centers advocate a diagnostic block with a local anesthetic, such as bupivacaine 0.5%, before neurolytic blockade; a favorable diagnostic block strongly predicts analgesia from neurolysis [37]. More recently, endoscopic, ultrasound-guided approaches that may prove safer and more cost-effective are being pioneered by gastroenterologists [38].

Evidence for the analgesic efficacy of celiac plexus neurolysis in intra-abdominal cancer pain syndromes is compelling. A recent meta-analysis of multiple retrospective trials and a single prospective trial found a high rate of successful pain reduction, regardless of malignancy type [39]. The results of 21 retrospective studies of 1145 patients characterized "adequate" to "excellent" pain relief in 89% of the patients during the first 2 weeks after the block. Partial-to-complete pain relief continued in approximately 90% of the patients who were alive at the 3-month point, and in 70% to 90% until death. Wong [40] reported on a prospective, randomized, double-blinded, placebo-controlled trial of patients who had unresectable pancreatic cancer, which compared neurolytic celiac plexus block and opioid treatment with opioid treatment alone and sham injection. Pain intensity was reduced in patients undergoing celiac plexus neurolysis, but a reduction in opioid and improvement in quality of life were not demonstrated. Reduced need for analgesic drugs and fewer opioid-related side effects, have been demonstrated in additional double-blinded, prospective, randomized trials [41,42].

The most common adverse effects of blockade are transient local pain at the injection sites, diarrhea, and hypotension [39]. Neurologic complications, including lower extremity weakness and paresthesia, occurred at a rate of approximately 1%, although paraplegia and transient motor paralysis have occurred after celiac plexus block [43]. A meta-analysis by Eisenberg and colleagues [39] found nonneurologic complications such as pneumothorax, pleuritic chest pain, hiccoughing, or hematuria occurring at a rate of about 1%.

Intercostal nerve block

Intercostal neuralgia following thoracotomy

Chronic chest wall pain caused by postthoracotomy, intercostal neuralgia, as a cause of direct neural invasion of a tumor, is difficult to control. Poorly controlled perioperative pain appears to be a risk factor for this form of chronic neuropathic pain [44,45]. Temporary intercostal nerve blocks have been studied extensively in a randomized, controlled fashion in the perioperative setting, and analgesic benefit has been demonstrated convincingly [46,47]. Postthoracotomy pain, which requires a multidisciplinary approach, is a common motive for referral to pain management clinics. The intercostal nerves are the primary rami of the thoracic nerves T1-T11. Beyond the midaxillary line, the lateral cutaneous branch of the nerve arises; the optimal location for the intercostal nerve block is at the posterior angle of the rib, lateral to the paravertebral muscles [48]. Much like other regional blocks that are useful in the surgical setting, the technical challenge with intercostal blockade is achieving durable relief.

The use of intercostal nerve blockade in the context of chronic pain has undergone limited study, with mixed results. One retrospective series of 123 patients found intercostal nerve block in combination with trigger point injection compared favorably with chronic opioid use in patients who had advanced cancer and prolonged postthoracotomy pain [49]. High-concentration local anesthetic (eg, 5% tetracaine), 10% ammonium sulfate, and alcohol have been reported in small case series for the treatment of this neuropathic pain [50,51]. Reduction in pain in these cases has far exceeded a block with local anesthetic, but long-term efficacy is unknown.

The most commonly reported complications are the extended spread of the local anesthetic or neurolytic solution into the root cuff, epidural space, and cerebral spinal fluid. This last effect can cause weakness and sensory loss in the blocked dermatomes. Moore and Bridenbaugh [52] have reported the rate of pneumothorax by radiograph to be 0.42% in the perioperative setting.

Spinal cord stimulation

Neuropathic pain syndromes

The strategy of modulating neural transmission with an electrical stimulus dates to ancient Rome with Scribonius' observation that the pain of gout could be alleviated through accidental contact with a torpedo fish [53]. Acceptance of the gate theory of pain in the 1960s led to renewed interest in electrical stimulation [54]. Gate theory proposed that pain perception was influenced by the balance of firing between small and large neural fibers. Retrograde stimulation of large fibers would provoke nonpainful stimulation, thereby "closing" the gate through adjustment in the level of voltage.

Shealy [55] implanted the first spinal cord stimulator for the treatment of chronic pain in 1967. In spinal cord stimulation, an array of stimulating metal contacts is positioned in the dorsal epidural space. An electrical field is generated through connection of the contacts with a pulse generator, and subsequently programmed in combinations of anodes and cathodes. The resulting field stimulates the axons of the dorsal root and dorsal column fibers, leading to inhibition of activity in the lateral spinothalamic tract and increased activity in the descending antinociceptive pathways [56]. Optimal stimulation is achieved when paresthesias overlap with the anatomic distribution of pain reported by the patient [57]. Either cylindrical, catheter-like leads are introduced percutaneously through a needle, or flat, paddle-shaped leads are deployed by way of an open surgical approach (eg, laminotomy or laminectomy). The power source, similar in size to a cardiac pacemaker, is implanted in a subcutaneous pocket and connected to the leads by way of subcutaneous tunnel. Advances in consumer electronics have resulted in more precise targeting of neuronal stimulation, improved battery life, and smaller device sizes.

Neuropathic pain of peripheral origin and ischemic pain states are currently the most common indications for this therapy. As with other interventional techniques, patient selection is the key to sustained efficacy. Pain associated with a lesion of the nervous system, or dysfunction, or so-called neuropathic pain, in a fixed distribution amenable to stimulation coverage, comprise the most basic requirements. Among the most commonly treated syndromes in the United States are chronic radicular pain after lumbar surgery and complex regional pain syndrome [58]. Neuropathic pain arising from lesions of the central nervous system does not tend to respond to spinal cord stimulation [59]. A temporary trial of stimulation, most commonly performed with percutaneous lead placement, is used to identify patients who might benefit from this approach. Accepted end points for trial stimulation include a 50% reduction in pain intensity, patient tolerance of paresthesias, global satisfaction with therapy, and reduction in analgesic medications [60]. The inability to blind patients to the stimulus of spinal cord stimulation in clinical trials, for preimplant assessment or evaluation of the benefit of permanent placement, is cited as an important limitation to the study of this modality.

Two prospective studies of spinal cord stimulation in complex regional pain syndrome have demonstrated a statistically significant reduction in pain intensity [9,61]. A study of 29 patients by Harke [61] enrolled patients with a prior response to blockade of sympathetic efferents (presumably selecting for subjects with sympathetically maintained pain) and demonstrated a greater than 50% reduction in Pain Disability Index scoring. Nearly 60% of these patients discontinued oral analgesic medications. An important technical limitation of this study was the high rate of battery replacement (55%) and lead revision (41%). A randomized study by Kemler [9] compared spinal cord stimulation and physical therapy in combination, to physical therapy alone. At 6 months and 2 years, the mean reduction in pain intensity in the spinal cord stimulation group was greater than 50%. At 3 years, the benefit of stimulation was waning, and a statistically significant benefit was no longer observed [62]. Alterations in neuronal connectivity, or neural plasticity, may account for this "tolerance." Three prospective studies in complex regional pain syndrome demonstrated a statistically significant reduction in VAS and a marked reduction in analgesic requirements [63–65].

Spinal cord stimulation is used as a late-stage therapy in the treatment of chronic radicular pain after lumbar and cervical spine surgery when other nonpharmacologic, pharmacologic, and less invasive modalities have not provided adequate relief. A prospective, randomized, controlled trial demonstrated superior outcomes with spinal cord stimulation, compared with lumbar reoperation [66]. Patients randomized to stimulation were less likely to cross over to the surgical treatment arm (5 of 24 patients versus 14 of 26 patients, $P = .02$) and required reduced amounts of opioid analgesics. The long-term reduction in pain intensity was reported at 50% in a large cohort of patients [67]. A low rate of technical complication in this study was attributed to the development of multichannel devices that appeared to limit the need for revision because of electrode migration. Progress in the treatment of the axial distribution of low back pain with spinal cord stimulation has been reported more recently in two prospective trials [68,69]. In these studies, the analgesic benefit appeared to be more stable in the radicular component. The evidence in another indication, refractory angina pectoris is primarily retrospective, but a recent trial demonstrated no advantage over percutaneous myocardial laser revascularization with regard to angina-free exercise capacity, and complications were higher in the stimulation group [70].

The most common complication of spinal cord stimulation across 15 trials (N = 531) was lead migration, which occurred in 18% [71]. Infection occurred in 3.7% of cases and battery failure in 3.3%. No studies in the above series reported epidural hematoma or paralysis, but there are reports of these complications.

Radiofrequency neurotomy

Facet-mediated spinal syndromes

Pain of spinal origin is the most prevalent chronic noncancer pain syndrome [72]. Providers disagree as to the role of particular anatomic structures and the underlying pathophysiology of low back pain [73]. The poor understanding of low back pain, lack of accurate diagnostic methods, and difficulty of designing studies to assess treatment efficacy have impeded therapeutic progress for this common problem. Interventional treatments that target specific structures rarely provide complete relief, but have been shown to alleviate symptoms when first-line conservative therapies such as medication, rehabilitation, and pharmacologic strategies do not reduce pain intensity and activity limitation. This section considers the evidence for one such intervention, radiofrequency ablation, to highlight the complexity and possible benefit of interventional approaches for the complex problem of pain of spinal origin.

The facet joint (or zygapophyseal joint) was localized as the possible anatomic source low back pain by Ghormley [74] in 1933. The facet joints are paired synovial joints formed by the inferior articular process of one vertebra and the superior articular process of the vertebrae below. A tough fibrous capsule is present on the posterolateral aspect of the joint. These small joints are supplied by the medial branch from the posterior ramus of the spinal nerve root. For much of the past century, interest in pain syndromes attributed to the spine's posterior elements has been overshadowed by radicular localization attributed to intervertebral disc herniation. Large-scale radiologic studies confirm that arthritic changes in these joints were common in asymptomatic patients and, therefore, not strongly correlated with the symptom of low back pain [75]. In 1963, Hirsch [76] showed that pain in the back and upper thigh could be produced by injecting 11% hypertonic saline in the region of the facet joint. By the 1970s, reports of treatment success with radiofrequency denervation of the medial branches revived speculation in the facet joint as a target for the treatment of cervical and lumbar pain [77]. More recent animal models have offered a biochemical basis for the movement-evoked pains attributed to the facet joint [78].

The diagnostic criteria for facet syndrome remain a matter of controversy. Older age, relief of back pain with recumbency, exacerbation of pain with extension but not flexion, localized tenderness with palpation of the region overlying the facet joint, absence of leg pain, and radiologic characterization of hypertrophied joints have all been proposed as relevant features of "facet syndrome" [79–81]. The lack of sensitivity and specificity of these signs and symptoms has complicated attempts to define inclusion criteria for treatment trials. Attempts to define facet syndrome through prospective study of intra-articular facet joint injection have not produced consistent, validated criteria [82]. Intra-articular injections with local anesthetic and steroid have proved to be of little value diagnostically or therapeutically for the treatment of chronic low back pain [83,84].

Review of the clinical studies of radiofrequency ablation for facet syndrome attests to the difficulty of assessing treatment efficacy in the absence of well-validated, diagnostic criteria. Two prospective, double-blinded, randomized, controlled trials of percutaneous radiofrequency neurotomy demonstrated lasting relief [13,85]. In these trials, patients were enrolled based on response to local anesthetic blockade of the medial branches or the dorsal rami supplying the putatively symptomatic joints [86]. The study by Lord and colleagues [87] achieved a minimum of 50% reduction in pain intensity for 263 days in the active treatment group with cervical zygapophyseal-joint pain after motor vehicle accident, compared with 8 days in the placebo group. This study applied an uncharacteristically rigorous protocol of three blocks (ie, two active, with differing concentrations of local anesthetic, and one sham block) to identify patients who had zygapophyseal joint (ie, facet) syndrome. Van Kleef and colleagues [85] replicated this result in the lumbar spine with patients selected by response to diagnostic nerve block of the posterior primary ramus of the segmental nerves at L3, L4, and L5. The primary end point of a 50% reduction in pain, or a more than two-point reduction on numeric rating scale, was achieved, compared with placebo in those patients with at least 1 year of chronic low-back pain. The patients undergoing radiofrequency ablation reported a reduction in opioid use and improved Oswestry Disability Index scores. A third small prospective trial and a large retrospective series (outcome assessed by third party) demonstrated prolonged benefit in patients with a positive response to diagnostic block, compared with nonresponders [88,89].

Much as in recent large trials of analgesics for neuropathic pain, the positive trial results characterized above must be considered in the context of a well-designed trial with a negative result [90–92]. A relatively large (N = 70), placebo-controlled, double-blinded trial by Leclaire and colleagues [93] of patients who had low back pain for more than 3 months, selected by positive response to intra-articular facet injection, did not show a benefit over placebo. The high placebo-responder rates in interventional trials may reduce the likelihood of demonstrating statistical superiority versus placebo, as has been observed in oral analgesic trials [94]. Others have suggested that the use of intra-articular block by referring physicians may have resulted in greater heterogeneity of the study population (ie, patients whose pain was not truly of facet origin). Such a view highlights the importance of precision in diagnostic injection techniques and interpretation, and the broader challenge of matching treatment to patient in chronic pain of spinal origin.

Minor complications from fluoroscopically guided percutaneous radiofrequency ablation have occurred at the low rate of 1% per lesion site [95]. Localized pain at needle entry site lasting more than 2 weeks was rare (0.5%) and there were no cases of new motor or sensory deficits in this series of 116 procedures (616 sites). Intrathecal injection has been reported in one case of chemical meningitis [96] and in a separate case of epidural abscess formation [97].

Summary

The patients who are candidates for interventional approaches are invariably those with the most severe pain. Locally-targeted therapy offers the possibility of improved pain control. These interventions do not supplant pharmacologic and nonpharmacologic modalities to treat chronic pain; their role is complementary. Intraspinal opioids, celiac neurolysis, spinal cord stimulation, and radiofrequency neurotomy all have demonstrated analgesic efficacy and the potential to reduce exposure to the systemic side effects of other therapies. The most challenging aspect of implementing these techniques is matching treatment to individual patient, and this is equally true of the many techniques not covered here. Diagnostic neural blockade with local anesthetics and temporary treatment trials of stimulation and intraspinal opioids enhance the likelihood of favorable outcomes. As the examination of intra-articular facet injection in low back pain reveals, placebo effect, a favorable natural history, and regression to the mean all may make it difficult to assess the actual benefit of interventions on a case-by-case basis. Experience is not a substitute for larger, placebo-controlled, randomized, prospective trials. Further advances await a deeper understanding of the correlation between symptoms and pain pathophysiology and a more precise understanding of the putative mechanisms of action of interventional therapies.

References

[1] Katz N. Role of invasive procedures in chronic pain management. Sem Neurol 1994;14: 225–35.
[2] Bonica JJ. Basic principles in managing chronic pain. Arch Surg 1977;112:783.
[3] Markman JD, Dworkin RH. Ion channel targets and treatment efficacy in neuropathic pain. J Pain 2006;7:S38–47.
[4] Rowbotham MC. Pain 2002—An updated review. Seattle (WA): IASP Press; 2002.
[5] North RB. Treatment of spinal syndromes. N Engl J Med 1996;335:1763–4.
[6] Block BM, Liu SS, Rowlingson AJ, et al. Efficacy of postoperative epidural analgesia: a meta-analysis. JAMA 2003;290:2455–63.
[7] Backonja M, Beydoun A, Edwards KR, et al. Gabapentin for the symptomatic treatment of painful neuropathy in patients with diabetes mellitus: a randomized controlled trial. JAMA 1998;280:1831–6.
[8] Lenzer J. Pfizer pleads guilty, but drug sales continue to soar. BMJ 2004;328:1217.
[9] Kemler MA, Barendse GA, Van Kleef M, et al. Spinal cord stimulation in patients with chronic reflex sympathetic dystrophy. N Engl J Med 2000;343:618–24.
[10] Burchiel KJ, Anderson VC, Brown FD, et al. Prospective, multicenter study of spinal cord stimulation for relief of chronic back and extremity pain. Spine 1996;21:2786–94.
[11] Boden SD, Davis DO, Dina TS, et al. Abnormal magnetic-resonance scans of the lumbar spine in asymptomatic subjects. J Bone Joint Surg 1990;72:403–8.
[12] North RB, Han M, Zahurak M, et al. Specificity of diagnostic nerve blocks: a prospective randomized study of sciatica due to lumbosacral spine disease. Pain 1996;65:77–85.
[13] Lord SM, Barnsley L, Wallis BJ, et al. Percutaneous radio-frequency for chronic cervical zygapophyseal-joint pain. N Engl J Med 1996;335:1721–6.
[14] Davis MP, Walsh D, Lagman R, et al. Controversies in pharmacotherapy of pain management. Lancet Oncol 2005;6:696–704.
[15] Mercadente S. Controversies over spinal treatment in advanced cancer patients. Support Care Cancer 1998;6:495–02.

[16] Mercadente S. Problems with long-term spinal opioid treatment in advanced cancer patients. Pain 1999;79:1–13.
[17] Enting RH, Oldenmenger WH, van der Rijt CDC, et al. A prospective study evaluating the response of patients with unrelieved cancer pain to parenteral opioids. Cancer 2002;94: 3049–56.
[18] Waldman SD, Coombs DW. Selection of implantable narcotic delivery systems. Anesth Analg 1989;68:377–84.
[19] Sjoberg M, Nitescu P, et al. Long-term intrathecal morphine and bupivacaine in patients with refractory cancer pain. Anesthesiology 1994;80:284–97.
[20] Hanks GW, de Conno F, Cherry N, et al. Morphine and alternative opioids in cancer pain: the EAPC recommendations. Br J Cancer 2001;95:587–93.
[21] Staats PS, Yearwood T, Charapata SG, et al. Intrathecal ziconotide in the treatment of refractory pain in patients with cancer or AIDS. JAMA 2004;291:63–70.
[22] Ballantyne JC, Carwood CM. Comparative efficacy of epidural, subarachnoid, and intracerebroventricular opioids in patients with pain due to cancer. Cochrane Database Syst Rev 2004.
[23] Smith TJ, Staats PS, Lisa TD, et al. Randomized clinical trial of an implantable drug delivery system compared with comprehensive medical management for refractory cancer pain: impact on pain, drug related toxicity, and survival. J Clin Oncol 2002;20(19):4040–9.
[24] Rauck RL, Cherry D, Boyer MF, et al. Long-term intrathecal opioid therapy with a patient-activated, implanted delivery system for the treatment of refractory cancer pain. J Pain 2003; 4:441–7.
[25] Kalso E, Heiskanen T, Rantio M, et al. Epidural and subcutaneous morphine in the management of cancer pain: a double-blind cross over study. Pain 1996;67:443–9.
[26] Kumar K, Kelly M, Pirlot T. Continuous intrathecal morphine treatment for chronic pain of nonmalignant etiology: long term benefits and efficacy. Sugical Neurology 2001;55: 79–86.
[27] Du Pen S, Du Pen A, Hillyer J. Intrathecal hydromorphone for intractable nonmalignant pain: a retrospective study. Pain Med 2006;7:10–5.
[28] Thimineur MA, Kravitz E, Vodapally MS. Intrathecal opioid treatment for chronic nonmalignant pain: a three year prospective study. Pain 2004;109:242–9.
[29] Emery E. Intrathecal baclofen: literature review of the results and complications. Neurochirurgie 2003;49:276–88.
[30] Smitt PS, Tsafka A, Zande FT, et al. Outcome and complications of epidural analgesia in patients with chronic cancer pain. Cancer 1998;83:2015–22.
[31] Grahm AL, Andren-Sandberg A. Prospective evaluation of pain in exocrine pancreatic cancer. Digestion 1997;58:542–9.
[32] Kappis M. Erfahrungen mit localanasthesie bie bauchoperationen. Verh Dtsch Gesellsch Chir 1914;43:87–9.
[33] Adolph MD, Benedetti C. Percutaneous-guided pain control: exploiting the neural basis of pain sensation. Gastr Clin North Am 2006;35:167–88.
[34] de Oliveira R, dos Reis MP, Prado WA. The effects of early or late neurolytic sympathetic plexus block on the management of abdominal or pelvic cancer pain. Pain 2004;110:400–8.
[35] Rumbsy MG, Finean JB. The action of organic solvents on the myelin sheath of peripheral nerve tissue-II (short-chain aliphatic alcohols). J Neurochem 1966;13:1513–5.
[36] De Cicco M, Matovic M, Bortolussi R, et al. Celiac plexus block: injectate spread and pain relief in patients with regional anatomic distortions. Anesthesiology 2001;94:561–5.
[37] Yuen TS, Ng KF, Tsui SL. Neurolytic celiac plexus block for visceral abdominal malignancy: is prior diagnostic block warranted? Anaes Intensive Care 2002;30:442–8.
[38] Abedi M, Zfass AM. Endoscopic ultrasound-guided (neurolytic) celiac plexus block. J Clin Gastr 2001;32:390–3.
[39] Eisenberg E, Carr DB, Chalmers TC. Neurolytic celiac plexus block for treatment of cancer pain: a meta-analysis. Anesth Analg 1995;80:290–5.

[40] Wong GY, Schroeder DR, Carns PE, et al. Effect of neurolytic celiac plexus block on pain relief, quality of life, survival in patients with unresectable pancreatic cancer: a randomized controlled trial. JAMA 2004;291(9):1092–9.

[41] Ischia S, Ischia A, Polati E, et al. Three posterior percutaneous celiac plexus block techniques; a prospective randomized study in 61 patients with pancreatic cancer pain. Anesthesiology 1992;76:534–40.

[42] Polati E, Finco G, Gottin L, et al. Prospective randomized double-blind trial of neurolytic celiac plexus block in patients with pancreatic cancer. Br J Surg 1998;85:199–201.

[43] Van Dongen, Crul BJP. Paraplegia after celiac plexus block. Anesthesia 1991;46:862–3.

[44] Perkins FM, Kehlet H. Chronic pain as an outcome of surgery: a review of predictive factors. Anesthesiology 2000;93:1123–33.

[45] Katz J, Jackson M, Kavanagh BP, et al. Acute pain alter surgery predicts long term post-thoracotomy pain. Clin J Pain 1996;12:50–5.

[46] Richardson J, Sabanathan S, Eng J, et al. Continuous intercostal nerve block versus epidural morphine for postthoracotomy analgesia. Ann Thor Surg 1993;55:377–80.

[47] Concha M, Dagnino J, Cariaga M, et al. Analgesia after thoracotomy: epidural fentanyl/bupivacaine compared with intercostal nerve block plus intravenous morphine. J Cardiothor & Vasc Anes 2004;18:322–6.

[48] Moore DC. Intercostal nerve block: spread of India ink injected into the subcostal groove. Br J Anaesth 1981;53:325–9.

[49] Moriwaki K, Uesugi F, Kusunoki, et al. Pain management for patients with cancer. Masui 2000;49:680–5.

[50] Doi K, Nikai T, Sakura S, et al. Intercostal nerve block with 5% tetracaine for chronic pain syndromes. J Clin Anes 2002;14(1):39–41.

[51] Miller RD, Johnston RR, Hosobuchi Y. Treatment of intercostal neuralgia with 10 per cent ammonium sulfate. J Thor Cardiovascular Surg 1975;69(3):476–8.

[52] Moore DC, Bridenbaugh LD. Pneumothorax: its incidence following intercostal nerve block. JAMA 1962;182:1005–8.

[53] Stillings D. A survey of the history of electrical stimulation for pain to 1900. Med Instrum 1975;9:255–9.

[54] Melzack R, Wall PD. Pain mechanism: a new theory. Science 1965;150:971–9.

[55] Shealy CN, Mortimer JT, Resnick J. Electrical inhibition of pain by stimulation of the dorsal column: preliminary reports. J Int Anesth Res Soc 1967;46:489–91.

[56] Linderoth B, Foreman RD. Physiology of spinal cord stimulation: review and update. Neuromodulation 1999;2:150–64.

[57] North RB, Ewend MG, Lawton MT, et al. Spinal cord stimulation for chronic, intractable pain: superiority of "multi-channel" devices. Pain 1991;44:119–20.

[58] Alo KM, Holsheimer J. New trends in neuromodulation for the management of neuropathic pain. Neurosurgery 2002;50:690–703.

[59] Villavicencio AT, Burneikiene S. Elements of the pre-operative workup. Pain Med 2006;7: S35–46.

[60] Windsor RE, Falco FJ, Pinzon EG. Spinal cord stimulation in chronic pain. In: Lennard TE, editor. Pain procedures in clinical practice. 2nd edition. Philadelphia: Hanley and Belfus; 2003. p. 377–94.

[61] Harke H, Gretenkort P, Ladleif H, et al. Spinal cord stimulation in sympathetically maintainted complex pain syndrome type I with severe disability. A prospective study. Eur J Pain 2005;9:363–73.

[62] Kemler MA, de Vet CWH, Barendse GAM, et al. Spinal cord stimulation for chronic reflex sympathetic dystrophy-five year follow up. N Engl J Med 2006;354:2394–6.

[63] Calvillo O, Racz G, Didie J, et al. Neuroaugmentation in the treatment of complex regional pain syndrome of the upper extremity. Acta Orthop Belg 1998;64:57–62.

[64] Ebel H, Balogh A, Klug N. Augmentative treatment of chronic deafferent pain syndromes after peripheral nerve lesions. Minim Invas Neurosurg 2004;43:44–50.

[65] Oakley J, Weiner RL. Spinal cord stimulation for complex regional pain syndrome: a prospective study of 19 patients at 2 centers. Neuromodulation 1999;2:47–50.

[66] North R, Kidd D, Farrokhi F, et al. Spinal cord stimulation versus repeated lumbosacral spine surgery for chronic pain: a randomized controlled trial. Neurosurgery 2005; 56(1):98–106.

[67] North RB, Kidd DH, Zahurak M, et al. Spinal cord stimulation for chronic intractable pain: experience over two decades. Neurosurgery 1993;32:384–95.

[68] Barolat G, Oakley J, Law J, et al. Epidural spinal cord stimulation with multiple electrode paddle lead is effective in treating low back pain. Neuromodulation 2001;2:59–66.

[69] North RB, Kidd DH, Olin J, et al. Spinal cord stimulation for axial low back pain: a prospective controlled trial comparing dual with single percutaneous electrodes. Spine 2005;30: 1412–8.

[70] McNab D, Kahn SN, Sharples LD, et al. An open label, single-centre, randomized trial of spinal cord stimulation vs. percutaneous myocardial laser revascularization in patients with refractory angina pectoris: the SPiRiT trial. Eur Heart J 2006;27:1048–53.

[71] Bennett DS, Cameron T. Spinal cord stimulation for complex regional pain syndromes. In: Simpson B, editor. Electrical stimulation and relief of pain, in pain research and clinical management. Amsterdam: Elsevier Science B.V.; 2003. p. 111–29.

[72] Andersson GBJ. Epidemiologic features of chronic low-back pain. Lancet 1999;354:581–5.

[73] Deyo RA, Haselkorn J, Hoffman R, et al. Designing studies of diagnostic tests for low back pain or radiculopathy. Spine 1994;19:2057S–65S.

[74] Ghormely RK. Low back pain with special reference to the articular facets with presentation of an operative procedure. JAMA 1933;1773.

[75] Magora A, Schwartz A. Relation between the low back pain syndrome and X-ray findings. I. Degenerative osteoarthritis. Scand J Rehabil Med 1973;5:115.

[76] Hirsch D, Ingelmark B, Miller M. The anatomical basis for low back pain. Acta Orthop Scand 1963;33:1.

[77] Rees WS. Multiple bilateral subcutaneous rhizolysis of segmental nerves in the treatment of intervertebral disc syndrome. Ann Gen Prac 1974;26:126.

[78] Toshihiko Y, Cavanaugh JM, et al. Effect of substance P on mechanosensitive units of tissues around and in the lumbar facet joint. J Orthop Res 1992;11:205–14.

[79] Jackson RP. The facet syndrome. Myth or reality? Clin Orthop Relat Res 1992;279:110–21.

[80] Lewinnek GE, Warfield CA. Facet joint degeneration as a cause of low back pain. Clin Orthop Relat Res 1986;213:216–22.

[81] Schwarzer AC, Wang SC, O'Driscoll D, et al. The ability of computed tomography to identify a painful zygapophysial joint in patients with chronic low back pain. Spine 1995;20:907–12.

[82] Schwarzer AC, Aprill CN, Derby R, et al. Clinical features of patients with pain stemming from the lumbar zygapophysial joints. Is the lumbar facet syndrome a clinical entity. Spine 1994;19:1132–7.

[83] Carette S, Marcoux S, Truchon R, et al. A controlled trial of corticosteroid injections into facet joints for chronic low back pain. N Engl J Med 1991;325:1002–7.

[84] Jackson RP, Jacobs RR, Montesano PX. Facet joint injection in low back pain. Spine 1988; 13:966–71.

[85] Van Kleef MV, Gerard AM, Barendse, et al. Randomized trial of radiofrequency lumbar facet denervation for chronic low back pain. Spine 1999;24:1937–42.

[86] Resnick DK, Choudhri TF, Dailey AT, et al. Guidelines for the performance of fusion procedures for degenerative disease of the lumbar spine. Part 13: injection therapies, low-back pain, and lumber fusion. J Neurosurg Spine 2005;2:707–15.

[87] Lord SM, Barnsley L, Bogduk. The utility of comparative local anaesthetic blocks in the diagnosis of cervical zygapophysial joint pain. Pain 1993;18:343–50.

[88] Gallagher J, Petriconne di Vadi P, Wedley J, et al. Radiofrequency facet joint denervation in the treatment of low back pain. A prospective controlled double-blind study to assess efficacy. Pain Clin 1994;7:193–8.

[89] North RB, Han M, Zahurak M, et al. Radiofrequency lumbar facet denervation: analysis of prognostic factors. Pain 1994;57:77–83.

[90] Backonja M, Glanzman RL. Gabapentin dosing for neuropathic pain: evidence from randomized, placebo-controlled clinical trials. Clin Ther 2003;25:81–104.

[91] Safirstein B, Tuchman M, Dogra S, et al. Efficacy of lamotrogine in painful diabetic neuropathy: results from two large double-blind trials [abstract]. J Pain 2005;6(suppl 3):S34.

[92] Thienel U, Neto W, Schwabe SK, et al. Topiramate in painful diabetic polyneuropathy: findings from three double-blind placebo controlled trials. Acta Neurol Scand 2004;110:221–31.

[93] Leclaire R, Fortin L, Lambert R, et al. Radiofrequency facet joint denervation in the treatment of low back pain: a placebo controlled clinical trial to assess efficacy. Spine 2001;26: 1411–7.

[94] Dworkin RH, Katz J, Gitlin M. Placebo response in clinical trials of depression and its implications for research on chronic neuropathic pain. Neurology 2005;65:S7–19.

[95] Kornick C, Kramarich S, Lamer TJ, et al. Complications of lumbar radiofrequency facet denervation. Spine 2004;29:1352–4.

[96] Thomson SJ, Lomax DM, Collet BJ. Chemical meningitis after lumbar facet joint block with local anesthetic and steroids. Anesthesia 1991;46:563–4.

[97] Alcock A, Regaard A, Browne J. Facet joint injection: a rare form cause of epidural abscess formation. Pain 2003;209–10.

THE MEDICAL
CLINICS
OF NORTH AMERICA

Med Clin N Am 91 (2007) 287–298

Invasive and Minimally Invasive Surgical Techniques for Back Pain Conditions

William Lavelle, MD[a],*, Allen Carl, MD[a],*,
Elizabeth Demers Lavelle, MD[b]

[a]Department of Orthopaedic Surgery, 1367 Washington Avenue,
Albany Medical Center, Albany, NY 122606, USA
[b]Department of Anesthesiology, Albany Medical Center, 43 New Scotland Avenue,
Albany, NY 12208, USA

Back pain is ubiquitous. More than 70% of people in developed countries experience low back pain at some time in their lives. Every year, one third to one half of adults suffer low back pain and 5% of people present to a nurse practitioner, physician's assistant, or physician with a new episode. Low back pain is most common in patients between the ages of 35 and 55 years [1,2]. In general, back pain can be attributed to a structural or neurologically mediated failure. Most cases of acute back pain are self-limited, with more than 90% of people recovering within 6 weeks; however, 2% to 7% go on to develop chronic, and, at times, debilitating back pain. Back pain has a high recurrence rate with symptoms recurring in 50% to 80% of people within 1 year [3]. Looking at the epidemiology of back pain, female gender, older age, and lower socioeconomic status are associated with a higher risk for back pain. Lifestyle factors that predispose for back pain include lack of physical activity, obesity, and smoking [4].

Pain generators

There is a multitude of causes for low back pain. In a study evaluating the pathophysiology of back pain presenting to a primary care physician, 4% of patients had a compression fracture, 3% had spondylolisthesis, 0.7% had a tumor or metastasis of another tumor, 0.3% had ankylosing spondylitis, and 0.01% had an infection [5,6]. The overwhelming cause of back pain

---

* Corresponding authors.
E-mail addresses: lavellwf@yahoo.com (W. Lavelle); alcsar@nycap.rr.com (A. Carl).

0025-7125/07/$ - see front matter © 2007 Elsevier Inc. All rights reserved.
doi:10.1016/j.mcna.2006.12.001
medical.theclinics.com

remains nonspecific. It can be postulated that this nonspecific back pain is attributable, at least in some way, to the degenerative process of the spine.

Observing the natural history of spinal degeneration, one can witness a cascade of radiographic changes. Disc degeneration seems to occur first. The aging process causes progressive changes in the intervertebral disc composition similar to the changes seen in other aging tissues in the body [7]. These changes to the biologic structure of the disc influence the mechanical properties of the disc. Aged discs have decreased stiffness and strength. Aging also causes an accumulation of degraded matrix material that can impair the normal metabolism of the remaining cells within the disc [7,8]. Some of these changes may be seen on MRI as "dark disc disease" [9]. Despite the fact that age-related changes are unavoidable and are found regularly in the discs and joints of a patient who has back pain, a direct relationship between age-related changes and pain has not been proved [10]. Often, disc failure is the beginning of a domino effect in the spine. Loss of disc integrity often leads to lessened anterior stability. This decreased stability from degenerative discs causes ligaments to buckle and hypertrophy from exposure to excessive forces, including new torsion forces. Finally, the facet joints often degenerate with hypertrophy [11–14]. Because degenerative joints may or may not be painful, back pain may result from this cascade of failure. Encroachment of bone spurs into the foramen of the exiting nerve roots may lead to the potential for sciatic pain involving the buttock and leg. The areas of the degenerating spine may fail at different rates. If the anterior disc and ligaments fail at the same rate as the posterior structures (eg, facet joints), anterior subluxation of one vertebra on another may occur and produce spondylolisthesis. This, in and of itself, may be painful, but it also may lead to compression of the lumbar nerves in the cauda equina and result in spinal stenosis [15].

Physicians attempt to explain back pain with radiographic findings; however, there is not always a relationship between radiographic findings and pain generators [10]. The overlap in terminology that is used to describe different symptoms exacerbates the diagnostic dilemma and leads to an increase in confusion between referring physicians, consultants, and, ultimately, patients. The condition of neurologic leg pain or paresthesia carries the general term of sciatica. Sciatica can be attributed to several causes; in general, it is due to extrinsic compression of the fluid-filled thecal sac or intrinsic nerve conduction dysfunction. Pressure on nerve roots may stem from a herniated disc, stenosis, facet, or ligament hypertrophy. Nerve conduction dysfunction may be caused by epidural fibrosis, arachnoiditis, neurologic tumors, or scar; however, disc herniation or degenerative stenosis from the failing and hypertrophied vertebral structures remains the most common cause of sciatic pain [16–19]. Sciatica cannot be explained entirely by a pressure phenomenon; inflammation of the nerve root also plays a role. The nucleus pulposus contains material that can cause inflammation and excite nerve roots [20,21]. Along with discs and joints, muscles and ligaments also can suffer the ails of degenerative disease and inflammation, which make them potential sources of pain. Molecular biology and genetics have yet to yield conclusive information about the true etiology of spine-related pain.

Similar terms and definitions, based solely on radiographic findings, often confuse the referring physicians as well as patients. Spondylosis is defined as the age-related changes that are seen on radiographs, with disc collapse and resultant spur formation as the hallmarks. Spondylolisthesis is the resultant vertebral translation that may accompany the degenerative processes. More advanced imaging, such as MRI, has increased the confusion. "Internal disc derangement" (IDD) is another ambiguous term that is used by spine physicians. Coined by Crock [22] in 1970, IDD was used to describe a large group of patients whose disabling back and leg pain worsened after operation for suspected disc prolapse [23]. IDD was intended to describe a condition marked by an alteration in the internal structure and metabolic functions of disc that were believed to be attributable to an injury or series of injuries that may even have been subclinical [23,24]. Annular tears are believed to be the major manifestation or cause of IDD [23,25]. The diagnostic criteria for discogenic pain attributable to IDD are based primarily on discography, which involves injection of contrast into the disc center and evaluating its morphology on CT and plain radiograph as well as monitoring the patient for a pain response.

1. CT discography reveals an IDD (eg, annular tear).
2. Pain is reproduced on provocative injection of the contrast.
3. As a control, stimulation of at least one other disc fails to reproduce pain.

Facet joint degenerative changes follow the degenerative process seen with the disc. When pain arises from this area, patients often complain of greater discomfort with spine extension or hyperextension. Once muscles weaken, any position can cause discomfort. As a minimally invasive diagnostic and therapeutic modality, facet injections may be offered; however, the diagnosis remains a clinical one. Studies with a high level of evidence that examined the true efficacy of facet injections are rare [26]. One study failed to find a statistically significant difference at 1 and 3 months between patients who were injected with corticosteroid and those who received saline injections; however, at 6 months, the patients who were treated with steroid had a marked improvement in their pain that was significantly higher compared with controls. Cointerventions were more frequent in the group that received steroids; despite this fact, a small improvement in pain was noted [27,28].

Other similar-sounding terms that may act as causes of low back pain are "spondylolysis" and "concomitant spondylolisthesis." The posterior elements of the vertebra may be disrupted by a stress fracture of an area of the spine called the pars interarticularis. This spondylolysis also can lead to a slippage in the lateral plane (spondylolisthesis). Anatomically, the pars interarticularis is the lateral part of the posterior element that connects the superior and inferior facets. By definition, pars interarticularis means "part between the articulations." Repetitive flexion/extension and rotation lead to microtrauma at this junction, and, thereby, fracture. In the athletic adolescent, spondylolysis is one of the most common causes of back pain; it should be investigated by spot radiographs in this population. In one series of 100 adolescent athletes who presented with low back pain, 47% had spondylolysis [29,30].

Despite the fact that scoliosis is described classically as a painless condition, up to 30% of patients who have adolescent idiopathic scoliosis complain of back pain [31]. It seems intuitive that spinal deformity would alter spine biomechanics and lead to increased stress and degeneration, and, therefore, pain; however, two recent studies found no difference in pain scores between patients who had scoliosis and were treated with a brace or surgery and a control group [32,33].

How discs fail

Each vertebral level of the spine experiences numerous forces imparted from above and below. Put simply, repetitive mechanical loading, at least in part, is believed to cause intervertebral disc degeneration. This mechanical loading causes a disruption that affects the physical and biologic properties of the disc. The mechanical destruction is accompanied by a cascade of nonreversible cell-mediated responses that causes cell death. Cadaveric experiments and computer models showed how various combinations of compression, bending, and torsion can cause the morphologic features of disc degeneration, such as endplate disruption, fissure formation in the annulus, radial bulging, disc prolapse, and internal collapse of the annulus [34]. As the repetitive trauma continues, nucleus pulposus material is pushed slowly into, and, sometimes through, the annular ring of the disc. The added structural support and configuration of the posterior longitudinal ligament (which is diamond shaped) often deflects the protruded disc material to either side; however, central protrusions may be seen. This disc failure often develops as the result of additive microtraumas that patients experience in their daily lives.

As with most disease processes, one element of failure does not adequately explain all that we know about disc degeneration. Studies showed that as the disc ages, the number of blood vessels in the vertebral end plates decreases; most disappear by the third decade of life. The number of viable cells at the core of the disc also declines at this time [35]. The chemical structure and organization of the disc, including the collagen fibril organization, begin to change and eventually disappear [23]. Questions remain as to whether all of these changes are the predecessors to degeneration or if they truly are the result of the mechanical stresses described earlier.

Symptoms improve or resolve in about 50% of patients [36,37]. This may be due to a decrease in the inflammatory response or reabsorption of the material causing compression. Those who fail conservative measures, such as oral analgesia, physical therapy, epidurals, or nerve root injections for 6 to 12 weeks, may go on to surgical interventions. In 1983, Henrik Weber [38] prospectively studied 280 patients who were diagnosed with an L4–L5 or L5–S1 disc herniation. In the short-term, the group that underwent surgery had better outcomes than did the group that did not undergo surgery; however, the difference was not significant after 4 years. Bowel, bladder, and sex-associated symptoms indicate that the central sacral neurologic structures are involved, and the patient should be considered for more urgent surgical intervention on the basis of cauda equina compression.

Surgical treatment for painful sciatica

Walter Dandy [39] performed the first documented surgical decompression for a disc herniation. In the early 1930s, Mixter and Barr popularized discectomy and laminectomy for the relief of sciatica-type pain [40]. This surgical decompression involves removal of ligamentum and lamina. The surgeon then retracts the dural sac to access the disc material that is compressing the nerve root. Knowledge of the location of the exiting nerve roots in the surgical field and proper method of nerve retraction are necessary to perform this surgery safely. Because surgeon knowledge, skill, and experience vary, outcomes may vary as well. In the days of Dandy, Mixter, and Barr, patients underwent a much larger surgery, with a wide laminectomy and disc debridement. Over time, the size of the laminar resection has become smaller, and the soft tissue dissection has been minimized. A typical laminectomy is outlined in Fig. 1. It is hoped that minimally invasive techniques have decreased scar tissue formation and the incidence of iatrogenic instability. This has not been proved in well-controlled, prospective, randomized studies. The use of a microscope or loops has assisted with minimally invasive surgery. More modern adaptations involve the use of tube-type tissue retraction devices. The tubular retractor system uses sequential, telescoping soft tissue dilators to establish a soft tissue corridor through the adjacent paraspinous musculature to the interspace of interest. Once this corridor is established, a tubular retractor of appropriate length is placed over the last dilator and is secured tightly using a table-mounted flexible arm [41].

Microdiscectomy by any method has become the operation of choice; it results in decreases in hospital cost, postoperative pain, and days missed from work [42–46]. The prevalence of recurrent disc herniation varies, and it may be related more to surgeon skill than to choice of operation [43]. Specifically, studies showed no difference in the rate of recurrent disc herniation treated by open discectomy or microdiscectomy [47,48]. Patients who

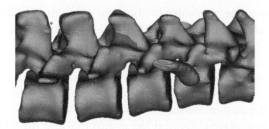

Fig. 1. A typical laminotomy for a modern discectomy.

undergo decompression have a more rapid resolution of symptoms; however, long-term results are no different when compared with nonoperative management.

Percutaneous discectomy, microscopic discectomy, tube-assisted discectomy (MetrX, Minneapolis, Minnesota) and energy-assisted discectomy Spine Wand (Arthrocare, Austin, Texas) are ways to minimize surgical exposure; however, minimal-access procedures require an even greater knowledge of spinal anatomy. Delineation of bone and nerve structures, as they enter and exit an operative field, is not possible with minimally invasive exposures. Better intraoperative imaging, such as computer-based image navigation devices (eg, BrainLAB System, Feldkirchen, Germany) may help with this challenge in the future.

Surgery for painful motion segments

As with other joints in the body, painful spinal motion segments may be treated by arthroplasty or fusion. We are just embarking on the frontier of spinal arthroplasty; none of the current techniques is considered minimally invasive. Fusion has been and remains the standard of care for a painful motion segment that failed conservative treatment. From the standpoint of fusion procedures, the evolution of care started with using local and harvested autologous bone to facilitate spinal fusion. These fusion techniques have been supplemented with structural support systems (eg, rods, hooks, wires, and screws). The advent of pedicle screws allowed for shorter fusion masses. Pedicle screws may be performed by a percutaneous technique or used to augment other percutaneous procedures.

Percutaneous pedicle screw placement begins with accurate identification of the levels to be instrumented. In a manner similar to performing vertebroplasty or kyphoplasty, 22-gauge spinal needles are inserted under lateral fluoroscopy in a paramedian approach so that they bisect the superior and inferior pedicles. The medial to lateral position of the needles is confirmed on the anteroposterior (AP) fluoroscopic image. Depending on the vertical distance between the pedicles, a skin incision that connects the needle sites may be made or small, separate incisions may be made at each needle entry point.

The needle is passed through the skin under fluoroscopic guidance. Once the bone is reached, the needle is advanced down the pedicle. Biplanar fluoroscopic images are obtained throughout the procedure. When the needle tip reaches the posterior vertebral body line on the lateral image, the medial pedicle wall on the AP image should not be violated. If the medial wall is violated, the surgeon risks intrusion of the pedicle screw into the spinal canal. A K-wire is placed through the cannulated needle, followed by needle removal. Sequential dilators are placed over the K-wire to develop a soft tissue corridor. The final dilator is left in place, and the pedicle is tapped under fluoroscopic guidance. Finally, a cannulated, polyaxial screw is placed over the K-wire, with the screw inserted under fluoroscopic guidance. Care is taken to avoid inadvertent advancement of the K-wire. This process is repeated for each screw.

After both screws are inserted, screw extenders are attached to the respective pedicle screws. The screw extenders are manipulated and mated. Rod templates are used to measure the correct rod length. A rod inserter is attached, and a separate incision is made at the site where a trocar will be placed to create the path of the rod through the soft tissues. The trocar is inserted until the most superior screw head is engaged. The trocar is removed, and the correct rod is inserted. The superior screw head is tightened, and compression or distraction is applied through the screw extenders. Finally, the rod inserter and screw extenders are removed [41].

Discs also may represent a painful motion segment. Posterior fusions alone may not alleviate pain at a particular vertebral level; anterior fusion may be necessary. Originally, this was performed through a second approach using an anterior or anterolateral exposure. This anterior exposure was popularized by surgeons from Hong Kong. The ability to accomplish similar stabilization procedures of the anterior column through a single posterior exposure would be a desirable next step. The posterior lumbar interbody fusion (PLIF), and, subsequently, the transforaminal lumbar interbody fusion (TLIF) approaches were soon popularized.

PLIF was performed first by Cloward in 1943. It was devised as a means to decompress nerve roots and perform a fusion procedure simultaneously [49]. Because his technique was not reproduced easily, it was abandoned until new spinal instrumentation and devices made the technique more viable [41].

The biologic advantages of PLIF include the elimination of an anterior approach, which itself, bears significant morbidity. From a mechanical standpoint, foraminal height is maintained, a well-vascularized fusion bed is created, and a shorter fusion distance is required [41,50]. Unfortunately, the preparation of the interbody region and placement of the device require significant nerve root retraction.

The PLIF technique may be applied thought two small paramedian skin incisions made at the level to be fused or in addition to a midline dissection that has been used for an open discectomy or decompression. The interlaminar space is accessed with any interposing soft tissue removed. Bilateral hemilaminotomies and medial facetectomies (Fig. 2) are performed, saving as much of the native bone as possible for the fusion. The traversing nerve roots are retracted medially, and a complete discectomy is performed. The endplates are prepared using decorticating instruments, such as rasps and curettes. The anterior disc space is packed with bone graft or a bone graft substitute (Fig. 3). Interbody devices, which may contain bone graft material, are placed. The fusion level is instrumented further with pedicle screws that are placed through the same midline or paramedian incision or percutaneously as described above (Fig. 4).

TLIF is similar to the PLIF procedure; however, TLIF was developed to address the concern of excessive nerve root retraction [41,51–53]. The TLIF device is inserted through a unilateral approach and theoretically minimizes nerve root retraction. Unfortunately, the approach does sacrifice a facet joint [41,50]. The TLIF device also may be inserted in conjunction with another decompression procedure or through an isolated paramedian approach. The proper level is identified, and the facet complex that is to be resected is approached surgically. As with a minimally invasive decompressive procedure, a tubular retractor system may be used to facilitate TLIF. A complete unilateral facetectomy is performed, with the resected bone saved for fusion procedure. Similar to PLIF, a complete discectomy is performed, and the interbody region is prepared again with rasps and curettes. After the area is prepared, the interbody is packed with bone graft or bone graft substitute. As with PLIF, the levels to be fused by the interbody device are instrumented with pedicle screws. The interbody device is placed diagonally across the interspace. The distraction across the interspace is released, and compression is applied. With all interbody fusions, one must be cognizant of spinal alignment. Loss of balance in the sagittal plane can lead to

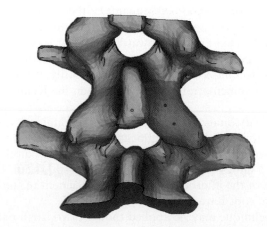

Fig. 2. The highlighted area illustrates the resection required for placement of an interbody device. The facet joint is removed, necessitating additional fixation (eg, pedicle screws).

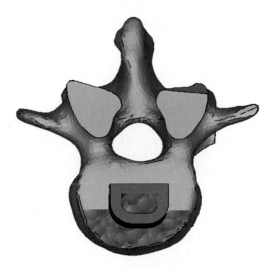

Fig. 3. Bone is placed within the anterior portion of the prepared interspace. An interbody device, which also may contain bone within its center, is placed.

a loss of normal contour, and, subsequently, to flatback alignment complications (eg, fatigue and back pain after standing for extended periods of time).

Problems with current imaging

Current imaging techniques are static images taken with patients in a recumbent position. When an individual feels pain, one typically is upright and performing an activity. Identifying areas for decompression may be difficult with this limited picture. Despite this, most spine surgeons believe that the current imaging studies are sensitive but not specific; therefore, a careful history and physical examination that correlates with the radiographic abnormality are imperative. Active images, such as forward flexion and extension radiographs, are used to identify aberrant and painful motion. Upright MRI imaging is becoming more popular; however, despite the logic that

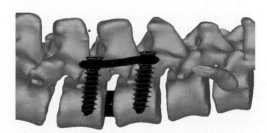

Fig. 4. Pedicle screws are placed to provide fixation across the interspace being fused.

patients should be imaged in the position that provokes pain, no well-controlled studies have substantiated this fact.

The need for physical therapy

If pain relief ensues following any spinal procedure or injection, conditioning and strengthening of the surrounding structures is necessary to allow continued pain relief and function. It is of the utmost importance to improve the debilitated state of the patient once the pain is improved. Physicians should have a low threshold for beginning physical therapy regimes for their patients. In addition, education about back pain is critical to its treatment. Studies showed that the patient's understanding of his or her pain significantly predicted treatment success [54–56]. Because most back pain is self-limited, the most minimally invasive procedure is always no procedure.

Summary

The treatment of spine-related pain is an ever-evolving area that requires a multidisciplinary focus. Our current fund of knowledge still relies on the decompression of compressed neurologic structures and the fusion of painful motion segments. Our approach for back pain management shows more attention toward biologically favorable decompression and fusion techniques. The future may hold a better understanding of the genetics and molecular biology of disc degeneration and facet disease, with the possibility of even more direct and less invasive interventions.

References

[1] van Tulder M, Koes B. Low back pain (chronic). Clin Evid 2006 Jun;(15):1634–53.
[2] Andersson GBJ. The epidemiology of spinal disorders. In: Frymoyer JW, editor. The adult spine: principles and practice. 2nd edition. New York: Raven Press; 1997. p. 93–141.
[3] Frymoyer JW. Back pain and sciatica. N Engl J Med 1988;318(5):291–300.
[4] Macfarlane GJ, Jones GT, Hannaford PC. Managing low back pain presenting to primary care: where do we go from here? Pain 2006;122(3):219–22.
[5] Koes BW, van Tulder MW, Thomas S. Diagnosis and treatment of low back pain. BMJ 2006;332(7555):1430–4.
[6] Deyo RA, Rainville J, Kent DL. What can the history and physical examination tell us about low back pain? JAMA 1992;268(6):760–5.
[7] Adams MA, Roughley PJ. What is intervertebral disc degeneration, and what causes it? Spine 2006;31(18):2151–61.
[8] Anderson DG, Li X, Tannoury T, et al. A fibronectin fragment stimulates intervertebral disc degeneration in vivo. Spine 2003;28(20):2338–45.
[9] Nissi MJ, Toyras J, Laasanen MS, et al. Proteoglycan and collagen sensitive MRI evaluation of normal and degenerated articular cartilage. J Orthop Res 2004;22(3):557–64.
[10] Battie MC, Videman T, Parent E. Lumbar disc degeneration: epidemiology and genetic influences. Spine 2004;29(23):2679–90.

[11] Garfin SR, Rydevik BL, Lipson SJ. Spinal stenosis: pathophysiology. In: Herkowitz H, Garfin SR, Balderson RA, et al, editors. The spine. 4th edition. Philadelphia: W.B. Saunders Co.; 1999. p. 791–826.

[12] Kirkaldy-Willis WH, Wedge JH, Yong-Hing K, et al. Pathology and pathogenesis of lumbar spondylosis and stenosis. Spine 1978;3(4):319–28.

[13] Garfin SR, Rydevik BL, Herkowitz H, et al. Spinal stenosis. Radiographic and electrodiagnostic evaluation. In: Herkowitz H, Garfin SR, Balderson RA, et al, editors. The spine. 4th edition. Philadelphia: W.B. Saunders Co.; 1999. p. 791–875.

[14] Troup JD. Biomechanics of the lumbar spinal canal. Clin Biomech (Bristol, Avon) 1986;1: 31–43.

[15] Leong JC, Luk KD, Chow DH, et al. The biomechanical functions of the iliolumbar ligament in maintaining stability of the lumbosacral junction. Spine 1987;12(7):669–74.

[16] McLain RF, Kapural L, Mekhail NA. Epidural steroid therapy for back and leg pain: mechanisms of action and efficacy. Spine J 2005;5(2):191–201.

[17] Cornefjord M, Olmarker K, Farley DB, et al. Neuropeptide changes in compressed spinal nerve roots. Spine 1995;20(6):670–3.

[18] Howe JF, Loeser JD, Calvin WH. Mechanosensitivity of dorsal root ganglia and chronically injured axons: a physiological basis for the radicular pain of nerve root compression. Pain 1977;3(1):25–41.

[19] Rydevik B, Brown MD, Lundborg G. Pathoanatomy and pathophysiology of nerve root compression. Spine 1984;9(1):7–15.

[20] Cavanaugh JM. Neural mechanisms of lumbar pain. Spine 1995;20(16):1804–9.

[21] Takebayashi T, Cavanaugh JM, Cuneyt Ozaktay A, et al. Effect of nucleus pulposus on the neural activity of dorsal root ganglion. Spine 2001;26(8):940–5.

[22] Crock HV. A reappraisal of intervertebral disc lesions. Med J Aust 1970;1(20):983–9.

[23] Zhou Y, Abdi S. Diagnosis and minimally invasive treatment of lumbar discogenic pain–a review of the literature. Clin J Pain 2006;22(5):468–81.

[24] Crock HV. Internal disc disruption. A challenge to disc prolapse fifty years on. Spine 1986; 11(6):650–3.

[25] Merskey H, Bogduk N. Classification of chronic pain: descriptions of chronic pain syndromes and definitions of pain terms. Seattle (WA): IASP Press; 1994. p. 180–1.

[26] Boswell MV, Shah RV, Everett CR, et al. Interventional techniques in the management of chronic spinal pain: evidence-based practice guidelines. Pain Physician 2005;8(1):1–47.

[27] van Tulder MW, Koes B, Seitsalo S, et al. Outcome of invasive treatment modalities on back pain and sciatica: an evidence-based review. Eur Spine J 2006;15(Suppl 1):S82–92.

[28] Carette S, Marcoux S, Truchon R, et al. A controlled trial of corticosteroid injections into facet joints for chronic low back pain. N Engl J Med 1991;325(14):1002–7.

[29] Lim MR, Yoon SC, Green DW. Symptomatic spondylolysis: diagnosis and treatment. Curr Opin Pediatr 2004;16(1):37–46.

[30] Micheli LJ, Wood R. Back pain in young athletes. Significant differences from adults in causes and patterns. Arch Pediatr Adolesc Med 1995;149(1):15–8.

[31] Sucato DJ. Spinal scoliotic deformities: adolescent idiopathic, adult degenerative, and neuromuscular in spine. In: Vaccaro AR, editor. Core knowledge in orthopaedics. Philadelphia: Elsevier Mosby; 2005. p. 137–56.

[32] Danielsson AJ, Nachemson AL. Back pain and function 22 years after brace treatment for adolescent idiopathic scoliosis: a case-control study-part I. Spine 2003;28(18): 2078–85.

[33] Danielsson AJ, Nachemson AL. Back pain and function 23 years after fusion for adolescent idiopathic scoliosis: a case-control study-part II. Spine 2003;28(18):E373–83.

[34] Adams MA, Bogduk N, Burton K, et al. The biomechanics of back pain. Edinburgh (UK): Churchill Livingstone; 2002.

[35] Trout JJ, Buckwalter JA, Moore KC. Ultrastructure of the human intervertebral disc. II. Cells of the nucleus pulposus. Anat Rec 1982;204(4):307–14.

[36] Weber H. Lumbar disc herniation. A prospective study of prognostic factors including a controlled trial. Part II. J Oslo City Hosp 1978;28(7–8):89–113.

[37] Weber H. Lumbar disc herniation. A prospective study of prognostic factors including a controlled trial. Part I. J Oslo City Hosp 1978;28(3–4):33–61.

[38] Weber H. The natural history of disc herniation and the influence of intervention. Spine 1994;19(19):2234–8.

[39] Dandy WE. Loose cartilage from intervertebral disk simulating tumor of the spinal cord. By Walter E. Dandy, 1929. Clin Orthop Relat Res 1989 Jan;(238):4–8.

[40] Wisneski RJ, Garfin SR, Rothman RH. Lumbar disc disease. In: Herkowitz H, Garfin SR, Balderson RA, et al, editors. The spine. 4th ed. Philadelphia: W.B. Saunders Co.; 1999. p. 671–746.

[41] German JW, Foley KT. Minimal access surgical techniques in the management of the painful lumbar motion segment. Spine 2005;30(16 Suppl):S52–9.

[42] Gibson JN, Grant IC, Waddell G. The Cochrane review of surgery for lumbar disc prolapse and degenerative lumbar spondylosis. Spine 1999;24(17):1820–32.

[43] Awad JN, Moskovich R. Lumbar disc herniations: surgical versus nonsurgical treatment. Clin Orthop Relat Res 2006;443:183–97.

[44] Andrews DW, Lavyne MH. Retrospective analysis of microsurgical and standard lumbar discectomy. Spine 1990;15(4):329–35.

[45] Barrios C, Ahmed M, Arrotegui J, et al. Microsurgery versus standard removal of the herniated lumbar disc. A 3-year comparison in 150 cases. Acta Orthop Scand 1990;61(5):399–403.

[46] Bookwalter JW III, Busch MD, Nicely D. Ambulatory surgery is safe and effective in radicular disc disease. Spine 1994;19(5):526–30.

[47] BenDebba M, Augustus van Alphen H, Long DM. Association between peridural scar and activity-related pain after lumbar discectomy. Neurol Res 1999;21(Suppl 1):S37–42.

[48] Toyone T, Tanaka T, Kato D, et al. Low-back pain following surgery for lumbar disc herniation. A prospective study. J Bone Joint Surg Am 2004;86-A(5):893–6.

[49] Cloward RB. The treatment of ruptured intervertebral discs by vertebral body fusion: indications, operative technique, after care. J Neurosurg 1953;10(2):154–68.

[50] Mummaneni PV, Haid RW, Rodts GE. Lumbar interbody fusion: state-of-the-art technical advances. J Neurosurg Spine 2004;1:24–30.

[51] Harms J, Rolinger H. A one-stager procedure in operative treatment of spondylolistheses: dorsal traction-reposition and anterior fusion (author's translation). Z Orthop Ihre Grenzgeb 1982;120(3):343–7 [in German].

[52] Humphreys SC, Hodges SD, Patwardhan AG, et al. Comparison of posterior and transforaminal approaches to lumbar interbody fusion. Spine 2001;26(5):567–71.

[53] Lowe TG, Tahernia AD, O'Brien MF, et al. Unilateral transforaminal posterior lumbar interbody fusion (TLIF): indications, technique, and 2-year results. J Spinal Disord Tech 2002;15(1):31–8.

[54] Henrotin YE, Cedraschi C, Duplan B, et al. Information and low back pain management: a systematic review. Spine 2006;31(11):E326–34.

[55] Deyo RA, Diehl AK. Psychosocial predictors of disability in patients with low back pain. J Rheumatol 1988;15(10):1557–64.

[56] Fardon DF, Milette PC. Nomenclature and classification of lumbar disc pathology. Spine 2001;26(5):461–2.

ELSEVIER
SAUNDERS

THE MEDICAL
CLINICS
OF NORTH AMERICA

Med Clin N Am 91 (2007) 299–314

Vertebroplasty and Kyphoplasty

William Lavelle, MD[a],*, Allen Carl, MD[a],
Elizabeth Demers Lavelle, MD[b],
Mohammed A. Khaleel, MS[a]

[a]Department of Orthopaedic Surgery, 1367 Washington Avenue, Albany Medical Center,
Albany, NY 12206, USA
[b]Department of Anesthesiology, Albany Medical Center, 43 New Scotland Avenue,
Albany, NY 12208, USA

The problem of osteoporosis

The aging population has brought new challenges to the medical community including osteoporosis, which is considered one of the most debilitating yet often ignored medical conditions. The National Osteoporosis Foundation estimates that more than 55% of Americans over the age of 50 suffer from either osteopenia or osteoporosis. Women bear the largest burden, making up approximately 80% of the affected population [1,2]. The hallmark of osteoporosis is fractures of fragility. A fragility fracture occurs as a result of a fall from standing height. The three sites that are typical of fragility fractures are the vertebra, hip, and wrist. Figs. 1–3 demonstrate a vertebral body fracture. With an annual incidence of 700,000, vertebral compression fractures occur more frequently than hip and ankle fractures combined [3]. Patients who have vertebral compression fractures often suffer such pain that it interferes with their daily living. Vertebral compression fractures account for 150,000 hospital admissions, 161,000 physician office visits, and more than 5 million restricted activity days annually [4]. In 1995, direct costs for osteoporotic fractures in the United States topped $13.8 billion, or $38 million daily [5,6].

Vertebral compression fractures frequently result in both acute and chronic pain, as well as leading to progressive vertebral collapse [5,7]. One thoracic vertebral compression fracture can cause enough overall sagittal kyphosis to cause a 9% loss of forced vital capacity [8–10]. Patients sustaining osteoporotic compression fractures also face increased risks for multiple

* Corresponding author.
 E-mail address: lavellwf@yahoo.com (W. Lavelle).

medical.theclinics.com

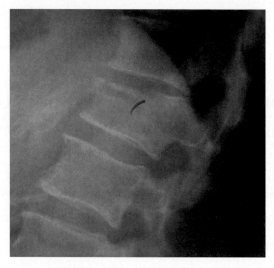

Fig. 1. A radiograph of a vertebral fracture is shown, demonstrating an osteoporotic compression fracture.

comorbidities such as weight loss due to early satiety and poor psychologic well being [11–14]. Although these fractures are rarely a direct cause of death, they do frequently produce significant morbidities that may eventually affect the mortality of the patient [12–19]. The 5-year survival of a patient who sustains a vertebral compression fracture is lower than that of a similar patient sustaining a hip fracture [12]. More commonly, elderly

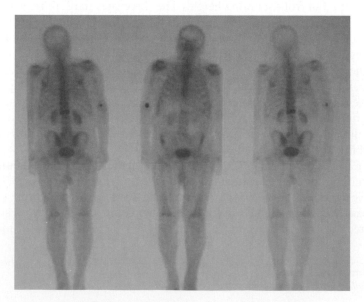

Fig. 2. Bone scan showing an acute vertebral fracture.

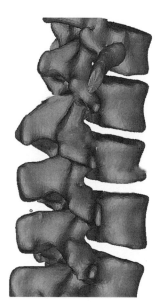

Fig. 3. Model showing a vertebral body fracture.

patients who were independent before their injury find themselves dependent on their adult children [20].

In the past, attempts at open surgical treatment of these injuries have been fraught with disaster. Poor bone quality would often lead to implant failure. Perioperative morbidity was often high because elderly patients bear other medical comorbidities. This has lead to patients being treated conservatively with oral, narcotic analgesia and an orthosis. Because this treatment offers little for those truly debilitated by their injury, physicians have become interested in new methods for pain relief and functional restoration to a degree that patients may return to their activities of daily living.

Use of cement in orthopaedics

Chemist Otto Röhm developed a new substance in the early twentieth century with novel structural properties and good biocompatibility. In the 1960s, Sir John Charnley began using Polymethyl methacrylate (PMMA) as bone cement on numerous patients for the fixation of both the femur and acetabulum for total hip replacement. Borrowing this idea from dentists of his era, bone cement acts as a grout, filling in the voids between the metal prosthesis and bone. [21,22].

In the spine, PMMA was first used to treat a painful and aggressive variant of a vertebral haemangioma [21–26]. Bone cement was later used to treat painful vertebral lesions caused by metastatic disease to the spine [27–29]. Multiple explanations have been offered for the pain relief associated with introduction of PMMA into an osteoporotic compression fracture site. Thermal necrosis and chemotoxicity of the intraosseous pain receptors have been offered as explanations in addition to the obvious improvement in mechanical stability offered by the bone cement [30]. It has been proposed that the cement monomer itself may be neurotoxic [31–33] and possibly act on the interossious nerve endings in the vertebral body. To create less viscous cement with a longer working time for use in percutaneous vertebral augmentation, more monomer is typically added to the powder than is recommended by the manufacturer [4,34,35]. The polymerization reaction of PMMA cement is exothermic. During the polymerization, temperatures can reach up to 122°C [36,37]; however, cadaveric study of osteoporotic vertebrae found that temperatures generated during vertebroplasty may not be sufficient to result in widespread thermal necrosis of osteoblasts [38–40] or nerve endings [41]. Whatever its mechanism, injection of bone cement into painful vertebral compression fractures is a successful technique with well-published clinical efficacy.

Indications for percutaneous vertebral augmentation

As with any surgical procedure, the typical patient who is offered percutaneous vertebral augmentation is one who has already failed several weeks of conservative therapy consisting of oral nonsteroidal medications and mild opiate analgesia. Usually, patients have been offered a supportive orthosis as well. The prime issue is mobility. Osteoporotic patients are at risk of significant medical morbidity the longer they remain immobile. However, controversy exists as to what the exact number of weeks or months of conservative therapy is appropriate before offering percutaneous vertebral augmentation. Some physicians offer an early percutaneous vertebral augmentation to patients who have a documented inability to mobilize after their injury. Typically patients who are mobile but still have pain are given 4 to 6 weeks to improve [5].

There are particular fracture patterns that are less likely to improve with conservative treatment, such as fractures of the thoracolumbar junction (T11–L2), osteoporotic burst fractures, wedge anterior compression fractures with greater than 30° of sagittal angulation, and patients with continuing radiographic collapse upon subsequent follow-up radiographs [5].

Despite the feeling that percutaneous vertebral augmentation is effective, the technique does have limitations and relative contraindications. Patients who have cortical disruption that would preclude cement containment should not undergo a percutaneous vertebral augmentation. Patients who have preexisting radicular complaints are often disappointed and report a poor result. This is perhaps because patients are undereducated about the difference between the subaxial back pain that would be attributable to the compression fracture site and the more peripherial radicular pain

that they are experiencing [5]. In the face of vertebra plana or complete vere-
bral collapse, any technique of percutaneous vertebral augmentation is difficult [42]. Obtaining preoperative imaging such as sagittal CT or MRI
images to assess trajectory and cortical integrity is often helpful [27,42,
43]. Bone scan may also be useful in determining fracture acuity because
these patients often have had previous fractures that may be obvious in
a plain radiograph but inconsequential in the patient's current clinical state
of back pain.

History of vertebroplasty

Galibert and Deramond [44] reported the first percutaneous vertebral
augmentation, or vertebroplasty. This landmark procedure was performed
in Amiens, France in 1984. These French physicians injected PMMA into
a C2 vertebra that had been destroyed by an aggressive hemangioma. The
authors reported that the procedure relieved the patient's long-standing
pain. PMMA was then introduced by way of a similar percutaneous technique aided by fluoroscopic guidance into the vertebral bodies of veterbra
that had sustained fractures caused by osteoporosis [45].

After the initial investigations in Europe, vertebroplasty was introduced
in the United States by interventional neuroradiologists at the University of
Virginia [46]. Veterbroplasty has gained increasing popularity with patients
reporting rapid pain relief [21]. The technique used to perform vertebroplasty has been modified with time to include larger bore needles and additional barium in the cement to decrease the risk of extravasation.

Technique of vertebroplasty

Before attempting a procedure on the spine, it behooves the practitioner
to have acceptable fluoroscopic imaging. It is the standard in the surgical
community to confirm the spinal level for the procedure with the patient
and the room staff. The procedure and level is again verified on the preoperative imaging and finally on the image intensifier before needle/cannula
placement. Proper imaging is essential to performing the procedure with
safety and precision. Proper cannula placement is observed on the fluoro-
scope before injection of the cement (Fig. 4). Fluoroscopic imaging also provides real-time images of the injection of the cement and the potential
extravasation into surrounding tissues, which represents the most likely
complication of the procedure [4,23,28,34,47].

As is done in many surgical procedures, prophylactic antibiotics are
administered to the patient approximately 30 minutes before the actual procedure; however, the efficacy of this practice in preventing infection has
never been affirmed by controlled study [4]. Some surgeons mix antibiotics
such as tobramycin into the cement that will be injected into the vertebral

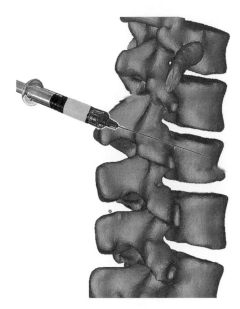

Fig. 4. For vertebroplasty, cement is injected directly into a fracture. The cement is injected under high pressure. The vertebral body is accessed through the pedicle.

body during the procedure; however, this practice is often reserved for the immunocompromised.

There are several anesthesia choices for percutaneous vertebral augmentation. Local anesthesia may be selected. The local anesthetic is injected in to the skin, subcutaneous tissues, and periosteum of the vertebra. Conscious sedation is often offered as an ajuant. General anesthesia is another possible choice. In cases that will involve CT guidance for needle localization, general anesthesia will best control for patient movement. General anesthesia is also the optimal choice for lengthy cases involving numerous levels of vertebral fractures.

After localization, a small incision is made and an 11-gauge cannulated trocar and bone biopsy needle is advanced to the posterior aspect of the vertebra. The cannula is passed through the pedicle into the vertebral body being treated. Both lateral and anteroposterior projections provide necessary visualization of the path of the needle. An alternative approach is a parapedicular. This is most often used to access the thoracic spine. The parapedicular approach involves inserting the cannula between the lateral margin of the pedicle of thoracic vertebrae and the rib head [23].

The most common approach involves accessing and injecting cement through both pedicles [23]. A unipedicular approach may also be employed. This approach does require a more oblique route because of the need to introduce the cement into the midline and anterior third of the vertebral body. The needle can be steered within the bone to allow injection into both sides of the injured body because of the beveled design [23]. Before injection of the

cement, a vertebrogram may be performed to identify the basivertebral venous plexus and other large vessels that are susceptible for extravasation
[48–50]. However this is often unnecessary, and in fractures that involve
the endplate, the contrast material may leak into the disk and not drain.
The remaining dye will mimic the contrast in the cement and preclude detec-
tion of cement leakage [48–50].

With single-plane fluoroscopic equipment, actual injection of the cement
should be visualized with lateral fluoroscopy [23]. Anteroposterior images
are checked regularly to monitor for lateral leaks. Deramond and colleagues
[4] suggest that all the cements available currently do not contain enough
barium sulfate for opacification on fluoroscopy; therefore approximately
30% wt/vol of pure barium sulfate may be added to the PMMA powder
before mixing and injection. Biplane fluoroscopy will allow simultaneous
visualization in two projections during injection. It allows the procedure
to be performed more rapidly [51] and is often chosen when the procedure
is performed in a radiology department because of equipment availability
and familiarity. CT guidance has also been described [52], but often adds
more to the cost of the procedure and has not become a popular adjuvant.
It is useful in the anterolateral approach to the cervical spine where the
carotid vessels must be avoided. It is also helpful down to the level of T4
where the shoulders will not allow for easy lateral fluoroscopy [52]. CT
and MR imaging limit real-time monitoring, and many surgeons will use
these modalities for placement of the needle and then use fluoroscopy during
injection [4]. Typically the injection must be completed in 6 to 8 minutes and
before the cement becomes too viscous to allow reinsertion of the stylus.
Otherwise a "needle cast" or a "cement tail" may remain in the soft tissue
as the needle is removed with the adherent cement [23].

The cement will set within 20 minutes and achieve 90% of its strength
within an hour [4,23]. Patients can typically sit up and walk once they
have recovered from anesthesia. On an outpatient basis, the patient should
be observed for 1 to 3 hours postoperation. Pain relief is expected to be
noticed in 4 to 24 hours. Clinical follow-up includes pain scale testing. Ra-
diography is indicated if the patient fails to respond positively to the intervention because an incorrect level may have been treated or a new fracture
may have occurred after the vertebroplasty procedure [3].

Results of vertebroplasty

Overall, vertebroplasty has been effective in relieving the back pain caused
by vertebral compression fractures. Grados and colleagues [53] assessed pain
relief with the use of the visual analog scale; they discovered a significant decrease in pain from 80 mm to 37 mm in just 1 month following the procedure.
The improvement was stable with an average assessment of pain at 34 mm on
the scale at a mean follow-up of 2 years. Zoarski and colleagues [54] at just 2
weeks follow-up also found significant improvement in pain and disability,

physical function, and even mental function as reported by patients. Of the 23 patients treated, 22 reported satisfaction at 15 to 18 months following verte-broplasty. In a larger group of 75 patients, Kaufmann and colleagues [55] found positive effects of the procedure with regard to pain measurement, mo-bility, and the use of analgesics. However, they did find that the procedure was less effective in patients requiring narcotics for pain control before the opera-tion and in those with longstanding fractures. Additionally, some reports have suggested a failure rate of up to 10%. Deramond and colleagues [56] suggest that failure rates much higher than this may indicate a flaw in patient selection; radiologists and clinicians should work as a team to select patients that stand to benefit the most from such procedures. These significant improvements re-sult from a procedure that does not attempt to reduce the actual fracture, but only stabilizes it.

As would be expected with any surgical intervention, vertebroplasty is not without its risks. Complications may be medical, problems with anesthe-sia, and instrument misplacement or technical error. Unique complications to vertebroplasty and kyphoplasty include cement extravasation and frac-ture of vertebral bodies adjacent to the levels treated.

Grados and colleagues [53] suggest a rate of cement extravasation of 6% for vertebral level treated with vertebroplasty. Rates of neural compression from such leakage may range from 0% to 4% [5]. However, in cases of true vertebral compression fractures due to osteoporosis, the rate may be lower within the range. Treatment for angiomas and bone metastases tend to have a higher rate of this specific complication—as high as 10% in some reports [56]. Specific technical safeguards and the use of contrast within the cement mixture are ways to prevent the most frequent complication of percutaneous vertebral augmentation.

History of kyphoplasty

The possibility of injecting highly viscous cement into fractured trabecu-lar bone was worrisome to spine surgeons. The fear that cement extravasa-tion could have devastating neurologic consequences from intrusion was of particular concern. Spine surgeons were also concerned that the high pres-sures used to introduce the cement could potentially lead to the bolus embo-lization of cement through the venous channels in the vertebral bodies to the lungs. Additionally, vertebroplasty was felt to be an inadequate means of fracture reduction. As a solution to all these concerns, the kyphoplasty tech-nique was devised and was first performed in 1998 [15,57]. The procedure seemed to result in the same type of pain relief.

Technique of kyphoplasty

All patients who undergo the procedure in our facility are anesthetized with general anesthesia. This form of anesthesia is chosen because the elderly patients in our population do not tolerate the prone position. The patients were prepared and draped in a normal sterile fashion. Fluoroscopic guidance is used to identify the fracture site to be treated.

A 1-cm incision is made just lateral to both pedicles of the vertebral body to be treated. A Jamshidi needle (Kyphon, Sunnyvale, California) is used to enter the superior lateral border of the pedicle under fluoroscopic guidance. Using a combination of manual pressure and light malleting, the Jamshidi needle is passed through the pedicle into the vertebral body. Frequent anteroposterior and lateral fluoroscopic images are used to confirm position. Once the Jamshidi needle enters the vertebral body, the needle is exchanged for an obturator (Kyphon, Sunnyvale, California) followed by a working cannula (Kyphon, Sunnyvale, California). A drill is then used to create a tract into the vertebral body. The balloon catheter is introduced into the fracture site and the process is repeated on the contralateral side. Both balloon tamps (Kyphon, Sunnyvale, California) are then inflated until either the fracture is reduced or it is felt unsafe to continue (PSIO300 or violation of one of the vertebral end plates). The balloons are then removed, and the cavities are filled with methyl methacrylate cement using a hand plunger system supplied by the manufacturer. Intraoperative radiographs are used to confirm containment of the cement in the vertebral body (Figs. 5–7) [3].

Results of kyphoplasty

Height restoration/fracture reduction

As one of the proposed device advances, fracture reduction results have been examined by several investigators. Within the confines of these studies, pre- and postprocedure images were reviewed to determine the degree of fracture reduction, particularly the restoration of vertebral height. Height restoration is determined by comparing the fractured vertebra to the adjacent vertebral segments.

Majd and colleagues [58] found in their series of 360 kyphoplasty procedures performed on 222 patients, a 30%-anterior fracture reduction or return of the relative anterior height was achieved. This study also looked at restoration of medial vertebral height; this restoration averaged 50%. Kyphotic angle was also examined, which is a relative measure that looks at how far forward a fracture causes a patient to bend as compared with the normal vertebral alignment. The average relative correction of the kyphotic angle was 7 degrees.

Boszczyk and colleagues [59] found a similar average correction of the kyphotic angle of 5 degrees with kyphoplasty. Within this study, a head-to-head comparison was made with vertebroplasty. No correction of the kyphotic angle was achieved through introduction of cement alone without use of a balloon tamp.

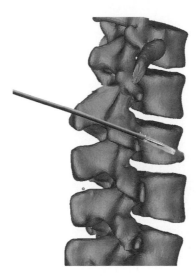

Fig. 5. For kyphoplasty, a balloon tamp is inserted into the fracture before cement injection.

Lieberman and colleagues [60] at the Cleveland Clinic reported on 30 patients who underwent 70 kyphoplasty procedures. Height restoration was again examined. When examining height restoration of the vertebral body as a whole, 35% of the relative height was restored in this series. With regard to correction of the kyphotic angle, a similar 6° of correction was achieved.

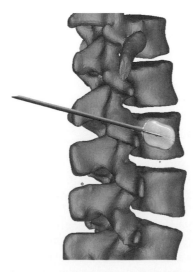

Fig. 6. An inflated balloon creates a void for the low-pressure injection of cement. Some feel the tamp acts as an aide for fracture reduction.

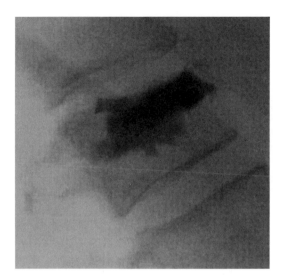

Fig. 7. Postkyphoplasty radiograph.

Crandall and colleagues [61] found the greatest degree of height correction at 86% in what were termed as "new" or acute fractures. Fractures that were subacute (older than 4 months) a 79% correction was achieved. The kyphotic angle correction differed based on fracture age as well. Kyphoplasty of new fractures resulted in a 7° correction whereas subacute fractures were reduced by 5°.

The most recent study by Pradhan and colleagues [8] was a retrospective study of 65 patients who underwent one- to three-level kyphoplasty procedures. Measurements revealed that kyphoplasty reduced local kyphotic deformity at the fractured vertebra by an average of 7.3°. Overall angular correction decreased to 2.4° (20% of preoperative kyphosis at fractured level) when measured one level above and below. The angular correction further decreased to 1.5° and 1.0° (13% and 8% of preoperative kyphosis at fractured level), respectively, at spans of two and three levels above and below. With multilevel kyphoplasty procedures, the total gains seen over multiple vertebrae, such as 7.8° over two levels and 7.7° over three levels, compared with the 7.3° for a single level. In other words, the small correction in fracture height and angulation achieved through the use of kyphoplasty does not translate into a substantial improvement in the general sagital alignment of the spine as a whole.

All of these studies have examined fracture by way of pre- and postop imaging. Reduction of the fracture through positioning in hyperextension may achieve a degree of fracture reduction. This explanation has been proposed as the primary means of fracture reduction by some spine surgeons. However, if this were an effective means of osteoporotic fracture reduction, better fracture reduction results with vertebroplasty would have been noted in the literature.

Pain relief

The first report on the kyphoplasty procedure was published by Garfin and colleagues [15] in 2001. This group found that 95% of patients treated with kyphoplasty or vertebroplasty had significant improvement in pain. Lieberman and colleagues [60] published the results of a phase I study of the inflatable bone tamp used in the kyphoplasty procedure. Seventy kyphoplasty procedures were studied in 30 patients. Pain scores improved significantly as a result of the procedure from 11.6 to 58.7 ($P = .0001$). Physical function scores also demonstrated significant improvement. In 2003, Ledlie and Renfro [62] followed 133 kyphoplasty patients for 1 year. These patients realized a reduction in visual analog pain scores from an average of 8.6/10 preprocedure to 1.6/10 postprocedure. Thirty-five percent reported unassisted preprocedure ambulation, whereas 90% reported unassisted postprocedure ambulation. In a separate multicenter study, 90% of patients treated by kyphoplasty were able to return to their baseline activities with 90% also able to wean off narcotic medications [15].

Risk of another fracture after percutaneous vertebral augmentation

Much speculation and concern has been raised about recurrent vertebral compression fracture, particularly at adjacent levels [3,63–70]. Unfortunately, patients who experience one osteoporotic fracture have a high likelihood of sustaining a second fragility fracture [71,72]. There are few reports that are available in the literature describing the actual incidence of another fracture after a kyphoplasty procedure [58,68,70,72,73]. In one review by Fribourg and colleagues [68], 17 additional fractures occurred after 47 levels were treated by kyphoplasty. Another study by Majd and colleagues [58] found an overall recurrent fracture rate of 10% (36 additional fractures in 360 fractures treated). Finally, the recurrent fracture rate published by Lavelle and Cheney [3] was 15% overall (16 of 109 treated levels) and 10% at 90 days. It seems from the literature that the incidence of a fracture after percutaneous vertebral augmentation falls within the realm of the incidence of a patient sustaining an additional veretebral fracture after a prior fracture. Although the incidence of a first-time vertebral fracture is 3.6%, the subsequent fracture rate may be as high as 19.2% within the first year [71].

Summary

Percutaneous veretebral augmentation offers a minimally invasive approach to a painful osteoporotic vertebral compression fracture. Both methods allow for the introduction of bone cement in to the fracture site with clinical results indicating substantial pain relief in approximately 90% of patients. Kyphoplasty offers the possibility of lower pressures for cement introduction and the possibility of modest fracture reductions.

References

[1] Lemke DM. Vertebroplasty and kyphoplasty for treatment of painful osteoporotic compression fractures. J Am Acad Nurse Pract 2005;17(7):268–76.

[2] National Osteoporosis Foundation. 2005 Annual Report. Available at: http://www.nof.org/aboutnof/2005_Annual_Report_FINAL.pdf. Accessed December 20, 2006.

[3] Lavelle WF, Cheney R. Recurrent fracture after vertebral kyphoplasty. Spine J 2006;6(5): 488–93.

[4] Mathis JM, Barr JD, Belkoff SM, et al. Percutaneous vertebroplasty: a developing standard of care for vertebral compression fractures. AJNR Am J Neuroradiol 2001;22(2):373–81.

[5] Truumees E, Hilibrand A, Vaccaro AR. Percutaneous vertebral augmentation. Spine J 2004; 4(2):218–29.

[6] Michigan Department of Community Health. Michigan osteoporosis strategic plan. Available at: http://www.michigan.gov/documents/osteorpt_6772_7.pdf. Accessed December 20, 2006.

[7] Wasnich U. Vertebral fracture epidemiology. Bone 1996;18:1791–6.

[8] Pradhan BB, Bae HW, Kropf MA, et al. Kyphoplasty reduction of osteoporotic vertebral compression fractures: correction of local kyphosis versus overall sagittal alignment. Spine 2006;31(4):435–41.

[9] Schlaich C, Minne HW, Bruckner T, et al. Reduced pulmonary function in patients with spinal osteoporotic fractures. Osteoporos Int 1998;8(3):261–7.

[10] Leech JA, Dulberg C, Kellie S, et al. Relationship of lung function to severity of osteoporosis in women. Am Rev Respir Dis 1990;141(1):68–71.

[11] Leidig-Bruckner G, Minne HW, Schlaich C, et al. Clinical grading of spinal osteoporosis: quality of life components and spinal deformity in women with chronic low back pain and women with vertebral osteoporosis. J Bone Miner Res 1997;12(4):663–75.

[12] Kado DM, Duong T, Stone KL, et al. Incident vertebral fractures and mortality in older women: a prospective study. Osteoporos Int 2003;14(7):589–94.

[13] Jalava T, Sarna S, Pylkkanen L, et al. Association between vertebral fracture and increased mortality in osteoporotic patients. J Bone Miner Res 2003;18(7):1254–60.

[14] Silverman SL, Delmas PD, Kulkarni PM, et al. Comparison of fracture, cardiovascular event, and breast cancer rates at 3 years in postmenopausal women with osteoporosis. J Am Geriatr Soc 2004;52(9):1543–8.

[15] Garfin SR, Yuan HA, Reiley MA. New technologies in spine: kyphoplasty and vertebroplasty for the treatment of painful osteoporotic compression fractures. Spine 2001;26(14): 1511–5.

[16] Cooper C, Atkinson EJ, Jacobsen SJ, et al. Population-based study of survival after osteoporotic fractures. Am J Epidemiol 1993;137:1001–5.

[17] Ismail AA, O'Neill TW, Cooper C, et al. Mortality associated with vertebral deformity in men and women: results from the European Prospective Osteoporosis Study (EPOS). Osteoporos Int 1998;8:291–7.

[18] Ensrud K, Thompson D, Cauley J, et al. Prevalent vertebral deformities predict mortality and hospitalization in older women with low bone mass. J Am Geriatr Soc 2000;48:241–9.

[19] Cauley JA, Thompson DE, Ensrud KC, et al. Risk of mortality following clinical fractures. Osteoporos Int 2000;11:556–61.

[20] Garfin SR, Reilley MA. Minimally invasive treatment of osteoporotic vertebral body compression fractures. Spine J 2002;2(1):76–80.

[21] Mathis JM, Maroney M, Fenton DC, et al. Evaluation of bone cements for use in percutaneous vertebroplasty [abstract]. In: Proceedings of the 13th Annual Meeting of the North American Spine Society (San Francisco, CA, October 28–31, 1998). Rosemont (IL): North American Spine Society; 1998:210–1.

[22] DiMaio FR. The science of bone cement: a historical review. Orthopedics 2002;25(12): 1399–407.

[23] Hide IG, Gangi A. Percutaneous vertebroplasty: history, technique and current perspectives. Clin Radiol 2004;59:461–7.

[24] Cortet B, Cotten A, Deprez X, et al. Value of vertebroplasty combined with surgical decompression in the treatment of aggressive spinal angioma. Apropos of 3 cases. Rev Rhum Ed Fr 1994;61(1):16–22.

[25] Ide C, Gangi A, Rimmelin A, et al. Vertebral haemangiomas with spinal cord compression: the place of preoperative percutaneous vertebroplasty with methyl methacrylate. Neuroradiology 1996;38(6):585–9.

[26] Feydy A, Cognard C, Miaux Y, et al. Acrylic vertebroplasty in symptomatic cervical vertebral haemangiomas: report of 2 cases. Neuroradiology 1996;38(4):389–91.

[27] Weill A, Chiras J, Simon JM, et al. Spinal metastases: indications for and results of percutaneous injection of acrylic surgical cement. Radiology 1996;199(1):241–7.

[28] Cotten A, Dewatre F, Cortet B, et al. Percutaneous vertebroplasty for osteolytic metastases and myeloma: effects of the percentage of lesion filling and the leakage of methyl methacrylate at clinical follow-up. Radiology 1996;200(2):525–30.

[29] Murphy KJ, Deramond H. Percutaneous vertebroplasty in benign and malignant disease. Neuroimaging Clin N Am 2000;10(3):535–45.

[30] Bostrom MP, Lane JM. Future directions. Augmentation of osteoporotic vertebral bodies. Spine 1997;22(24 Suppl):38S–42S.

[31] Dahl OE, Garvik LJ, Lyberg T. Toxic effects of methylmethacrylate monomer on leukocytes and endothelial cells in vitro. Acta Orthop Scand 1994;65(2):147–53.

[32] Danilewicz-Stysiak Z. Experimental investigations on the cytotoxic nature of methyl methacrylate. J Prosthet Dent 1980;44(1):13–6.

[33] Seppalainen AM, Rajaniemi R. Local neurotoxicity of methyl methacrylate among dental technicians. Am J Ind Med 1984;5(6):471–7.

[34] Deramond H, Depriester C, Toussaint P, et al. Percutaneous vertebroplasty. Semin Musculoskelet Radiol 1997;1(2):285–96.

[35] Jasper LE, Deramond H, Mathis JM, et al. The effect of monomer-to-powder ratio on the material properties of cranioplastic. Bone 1999;25(2 Suppl):27S–9S.

[36] San Millan Ruiz D, Burkhardt K, Jean B, et al. Pathology findings with acrylic implants. Bone 1999;25(2 Suppl):85S–90S.

[37] Jefferiss CD, Lee AJC, Ling RSM. Thermal aspects of self-curing polymethylmethacrylate. J Bone Joint Surg 1975;57B(4):511–8.

[38] Eriksson RA, Albrektsson T, Magnusson B. Assessment of bone viability after heat trauma: a histological, histochemical and vital microscopic study in the rabbit. Scand J Plast Reconstr Surg 1984;18:261–8.

[39] Eriksson RA, Albrektsson T. The effect of heat on bone regeneration: an experimental study in the rabbit using the bone growth chamber. J Oral Maxillofac Surg 1984;42(11):705–11.

[40] Rouiller C, Majno G. Morphological and chemical studies of bones after the application of heat. Beitr Pathol Anat 1953;113(1):100–20.

[41] De Vrind HH, Wondergem J, Haveman J. Hyperthermia-induced damage to rat sciatic nerve assessed in vivo with functional methods and with electrophysiology. J Neurosci Methods 1992;45(3):165–74.

[42] Cotten A, Boutry N, Cortet B, et al. Percutaneous vertebroplasty: state of the art. Radiographics 1998;18(2):311–20.

[43] Barr JD, Barr MS, Lemley TJ, et al. Percutaneous vertebroplasty for pain relief and spinal stabilization. Spine 2000;25(8):923–8.

[44] Galibert P, Deramond H, Rosat P, et al. Preliminary note on the treatment of vertebral angioma by percutaneous acrylic vertebroplasty. Neurochirurgie 1987;33:166–8.

[45] Bascoulergue Y, Duquesnel J, Leclercq R, et al. Percutaneous injection of methyl methacrylate in the vertebral body for the treatment of various diseases: percutaneous vertebroplasty [abstract]. Radiology 1988;169P:372.

[46] Jensen ME, Evans AJ, Mathis JM, et al. Percutaneous polymethylmethacrylate vertebroplasty in the treatment of osteoporotic vertebral body compression fractures: technical aspects. AJNR Am J Neuroradiol 1997;18(10):1897–904.

[47] Padovani B, Kasriel O, Brunner P, et al. Pulmonary embolism caused by acrylic cement: a rare complication of percutaneous vertebroplasty. AJNR Am J Neuroradiol 1999;20(3): 375–7.

[48] McGraw JK, Heatwole EV, Strnad BT, et al. Predictive value of intraosseous venography before percutaneous vertebroplasty. J Vasc Interv Radiol 2002;13(2 Pt 1):149–53.

[49] Gaughen JR Jr, Jensen ME, Schweickert PA, et al. Relevance of antecedent venography in percutaneous vertebroplasty for the treatment of osteoporotic compression fractures. AJNR Am J Neuroradiol 2002;23(4):594–600.

[50] Vasconcelos C, Gailloud P, Beauchamp NJ, et al. Is percutaneous vertebroplasty without pretreatment venography safe? Evaluation of 205 consecutives procedures. AJNR Am J Neuroradiol 2002;23(6):913–7.

[51] Wehrli FW, Ford JC, Haddad JG. Osteoporosis: clinical assessment with quantitative MR imaging in diagnosis. Radiology 1995;196(3):631–41.

[52] Gangi A, Kastler BA, Dietemann JL. Percutaneous vertebroplasty guided by a combination of CT and fluoroscopy. AJNR Am J Neuroradiol 1994;15(1):83–6.

[53] Grados F, Depriester C, Cayrolle G, et al. Long-term observations of vertebral osteoporotic fractures treated by percutaneous vertebroplasty. Rheumatology (Oxford) 2000;39:1410–4.

[54] Zoarski GH, Snow P, Olan WJ, et al. Percutaneous vertebroplasty for osteoporotic compression fractures: quantitative prospective evaluation of long-term outcomes. J Vasc Interv Radiol 2002;13:139–48.

[55] Kaufmann TJ, Jensen ME, Schweickert PA, et al. Age of fracture and clinical outcomes of percutaneous vertebroplasty. AJNR Am J Neuroradiol 2001;22:1860–3.

[56] Deramond H, Depriester C, Galibert P, et al. Percutaneous vertebroplasty with polymethylmethacrylate: technique, indications, and results. Radiol Clin North Am 1998;36:533–46.

[57] Armsen N, Boszczyk B. Vertebro-/kyphoplasty history, development, results. Eur J Trauma 2005;5:433–41.

[58] Majd ME, Farley S, Holt RT. Preliminary outcomes and efficacy of the first 360 consecutive kyphoplasties for the treatment of painful osteoporotic vertebral compression fractures. Spine J 2005;5(3):244–55.

[59] Boszczyk BM, Bierschneider M, Schmid K, et al. Microsurgical interlaminary vertebro- and kyphoplasty for severe osteoporotic fractures. J Neurosurg 2004;100(1 Suppl):32–7.

[60] Lieberman IH, Dudeney S, Reinhardt MK, et al. Initial outcome and efficacy of "kyphoplasty" in the treatment of painful osteoporotic vertebral compression fractures. Spine 2001;26(14):1631–8.

[61] Crandall D, Slaughter D, Hankins PJ, et al. Acute versus chronic vertebral compression fractures treated with kyphoplasty: early results. Spine J 2004;4(4):418–24.

[62] Ledlie JT, Renfro M. Balloon kyphoplasty: One-year outcomes in vertebral body height restoration, chronic pain, and activity levels. J Neurosurg 2003;98(Suppl. 1):36–42.

[63] Belkoff SM, Mathis JM, Fenton DC, et al. An ex vivo biomechanical evaluation of an inflatable bone tamp used in the treatment of compression fracture. Spine 2001;26:151–6.

[64] Villarraga ML, Bellezza AJ, Harrigan TP, et al. The biomechanical effects of kyphoplasty on treated and adjacent nontreated vertebral bodies. J Spinal Disord Tech 2005;18:84–91.

[65] Uppin AA, Hirsch JA, Centenera LV, et al. Occurrence of new vertebral body fracture after percutaneous vertebroplasty in patients with osteoporosis. Radiology 2003;226: 119–24.

[66] Polikeit A, Nolte LP, Ferguson SJ. The effect of cement augmentation on the load transfer in an osteoporotic functional spinal unit: finite element analysis. Spine 2003;28:991–6.

[67] Spivak J, Johnson M. Percutaneous treatment of vertebral body pathology. J Am Acad Orthop Surg 2005;13:6–17.

[68] Fribourg D, Tang C, Sra P, et al. Incidence of subsequent vertebral fracture after kyphoplasty. Spine 2004;29:2270–6.

[69] Berlemann U, Ferguson SJ, Nolte LP, et al. Adjacent vertebral failure after vertebroplasty: a biomechanical investigation. J Bone Joint Surg Br 2002;84:748–52.

[70] Cohen D, Feinberg P. Secondary osteoporotic compression fractures after kyphoplasty. Am Acad Orthop Surg. Meeting; February 5–9, 2003; New Orleans (LA): Poster no. P31.

[71] Lindsay R, Silverman SL, Cooper C, et al. Risk of new vertebral fracture in the year following a fracture. JAMA 2001;285:320–3.

[72] Kanis J, Johnell O, Oden A, et al. The risk and burden of vertebral fractures in Sweden. Osteoporos Int 2004;15:20–6.

[73] Harrop J, Prpa B, Reinhardt M, et al. Primary and secondary osteoporosis incidence of subsequent vertebral compression fractures after kyphoplasty. Spine 2004;29:2120–5.

THE MEDICAL
CLINICS
OF NORTH AMERICA

ELSEVIER
SAUNDERS

Med Clin N Am 91 (2007) 315–320

Index

Note: Page numbers of article titles are in **boldface** type.

Moving?

Make sure your subscription moves with you!

To notify us of your new address, find your **Clinics Account Number** (located on your mailing label above your name), and contact customer service at:

E-mail: elspcs@elsevier.com

800-654-2452 (subscribers in the U.S. & Canada)
407-345-4000 (subscribers outside of the U.S. & Canada)

Fax number: 407-363-9661

Elsevier Periodicals Customer Service
6277 Sea Harbor Drive
Orlando, FL 32887-4800

*To ensure uninterrupted delivery of your subscription, please notify us at least 4 weeks in advance of move.